REVERSE DEPRESSION NATURALLY

Alternative Treatments for Mood Disorders, Anxiety and Stress

Michelle Honda

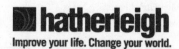

hatherleigh

Improve your life. Change your world.

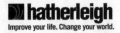

hatherleigh
Improve your life. Change your world.

Hatherleigh Press is committed to preserving and protecting the natural resources of the earth. Environmentally responsible and sustainable practices are embraced within the company's mission statement.

Visit us at www.hatherleighpress.com and register online for free offers, discounts, special events, and more.

Reverse Inflammation Naturally
Text Copyright © 2020 Michelle Honda

Library of Congress Cataloging-in-Publication Data is available.
ISBN: 978-1-57826-836-8

DISCLAIMER
Limit of Liability/Disclaimer of Warranty
This book contains nutrition and plant-based suggestions. The intention of this book is to complement a person's current treatment plan. The author recognizes a qualified physician or health care professional should be consulted regarding your specific complaint. The author does not recommend self-diagnosis or treatment. The publisher and author specifically disclaim any and all liability occurring directly or indirectly from the application of any information contained in this book.

Printed in the United States
10 9 8 7 6 5 4 3 2 1

Follow Michelle Honda, PhD on Facebook:
www.facebook.com/NewHopeForCrohnsAndColitis

To learn lots about nutrition and healthy living, and for more information on her private practice, visit Michelle's blog:
www.michellehonda.com.

CONTENTS

FOREWORD

by Sam Graci, H.B.A.

ALL LIFE-FORMS—FROM BACTERIA to bumblebees to tigers—share the same basic instincts. But humans are the only creatures on Earth with a big enough brain to make long-term decisions to support the goal of a happy, content, meaningful and purposeful.

Ironically, because we have such large neural networks, they can also get "overloaded," "malnourished," "stressed out" and literally "broken." And it happens to every one of us, from time to time!

Fire was one of the first tools humans discovered to better their lives. But today, the brain-exhausting fires of a never-ending flood of "to-do's", feeling mentally foggy, exhausted, disillusioned, slightly cranky—a case of the blahs—can stunt your creativity and curiosity, robbing you of a happy, and balanced brain.

The book you hold in your hands, *Reverse Depression Naturally: Alternative Treatments for Mood Disorders, Anxiety and Stress*, offers practical solutions to raise our happiness and satisfaction levels significantly. This powerful and easy-to-read roadmap tells us that somewhere in our brain's 100 billion neurons and 100 trillion connections are the neural codes that gave us *The Sound of Music*, Leonardo da Vinci's masterpieces and the futuristic cell phone you have in your pocket.

Luckily for all of us, our brain is as adaptable as it is complicated—and we are always getting better at biohacking it to rewire and restore optimal brain activity and function. Simple systems offer fewer entry points to intervene and take over their operation, but complicated systems offer many opportunities to upgrade, renew, restore and rejuvenate.

That is exactly how Michelle Honda presents her brilliant options to biohack your brain and quickly boost your physical performance and mental processing efficiency—naturally! And with your new-found good mood, you can be a smarter and brighter version of yourself with a more agile and resilient brain—all through natural tools that are closer than you can imagine.

That's the Michelle Honda promise—a radical new and natural plan for a vibrant, renewed, powered-up and happy brain.

—Sam Graci. H.B.A.,
    Ed Specialist, co-author of
    Love Your Life...Un-Com-Mon

INTRODUCTION

Worldwide, depression is spreading like a modern-day plague. The U.S. Department of Health and Human Services reports 1.7 billion people worldwide suffer from this mental illness; of those, more than 90 million are Americans.[1]

Regrettably, a large percentage does not receive appropriate mental health treatment, leading to widespread loss of function and drive. According to the Geneva World Health Organization,[2] depression is listed as the number one cause of disability throughout the world, with resultant economic losses exceeding one trillion dollars yearly. Suicide rates are also on the rise; since 1999, suicide rates have risen 24 percent in the United States.[3]

Something needs to change, and quickly, or these statistics will only continue to worsen as more and more people fall victim to the pervasive, crippling effects of depression and its related symptoms. Traditional treatment therapies are clearly insufficient to the task; if they were, we would not be seeing such a steep increase in life-changing symptoms, violent and suicidal behaviors, and death. In fact, there is some evidence to suggest that the widespread use of antidepressants and psychotic medication have contributed to this trend.

As you make your way through this book, you will learn about the different types of mental, physical and emotional imbalances that occur as a result of depressive mental illnesses.

You will also discover methods for normalizing both acute and chronic depressive symptoms and in doing so, you will be amazed at the number of related health complaints that diminish or disappear altogether with the management of your depression. People suffering with mood disorders are never without a collection of other complaints, such as fatigue, exhaustion, weight gain or loss, cognition impairment, insomnia, sugar reregulation problems, cholesterol imbalance, heart and circulation irregularities and sexual dysfunction…to name just a few.

This is because a healthy mind leads to a healthy body—and vice versa. When the mind is out of balance, the body will follow suit, leading to the laundry list of concurrent ailments described above. When the body spends a protracted period of time functioning at lower than normal levels, our system becomes nutrient-poor, or polluted; we don't have the energy and materials we need to perform normal bodily functions. This in turn builds a platform for disease and emotional imbalance, leading to the development of unwanted symptoms and illnesses, all of which are in turn supported by malnutrition and poor lifestyle choices resulting from a lack of drive to do better. This creates a vicious cycle, from which true escape can be challenging.

For a problem this complex and interconnected, there can be no magic pill! All aspects of a depressive disorder and its other health problems must be addressed; it is not enough to simply treat anxiety or a psychotic episode with mind-numbing drugs.

Within the pages of this book you will find natural, effective solutions to a myriad of complications surrounding depressive disorders. These remedies are provided with only one goal in mind—returning you to your whole, productive, happy self. In fact, you should expect to feel better than ever before—a return to an even happier self than before your first depressive symptoms were realized.

When embarking on the path less traveled, it is important to have faith in your own guidance system. Be patient; allow your body the time it needs to reinvent itself and embrace unfamiliar territory. Take the time to learn about the different types of integrative medicine showcased in this book, as well as complementary therapies and your body's biochemical nutrient requirements.

Likewise, learn more about any medications you may be taking or are prescribed to start. There are very real shortcomings and long-term unwanted side effects from the use of SSRIs and other psychotic drugs, all of which will be thoroughly discussed in this book. In fact, a main reason for the formulation of this book was to investigate the problems posed by the physical and emotional changes caused by antidepressant and psychotic drug protocols.

Understandably, you may find yourself looking for guidance as you try to replace or complement your existing medications and treatment plans with a more natural, whole body approach. To help accomplish this feat, we've provided step-step protocols to assist in alleviating all aspects of mood disorders, including protocols for strengthening a weakened and stressed mind and body.

The number one problem faced by patients attempting to get off of a psychotic medication or antidepressant is the initial return of their anxiety and other depressive symptoms. There need to be substitutes in place that can be called upon at will, to calm and provide relief no matter the complaint—without any harmful repercussions. This book also contains information on natural cures that can be relied upon to provide immediate relief, as well as general maintenance of symptoms.

This volume draws from my years of clinical experience and supportive research for the reversal of mental health outcomes, enabling you to confidently and effectively improve your personal health experience. It is my hope that you will find this book quite different from conventional medical treatment plans, with its strong emphasis on nutritional biochemistry, an intrinsic factor in the pathogenesis of mental health disorders.

The best news is that you will not need the natural drug substitutions recommended in this book indefinitely, even though they are safe, non-addictive and may be taken on an as-needed basis. It is primarily through nutrition and specific nutrient support that we will seek to restore the mind and body, creating a sound foundation for better health.

The only way a person can remain well or reverse their illness is by incorporating all aspects of the self—body and mind—in their treatment. But this process can only truly begin from a place of understanding and commitment. It is my hope that this book provides the information you need to help you break the cycle of symptom and medication, and regain your independence, your drive, and your hope for the future.

—Michelle Honda Ph.D. D.Sc.

CHAPTER 1

Depression: A Modern Day Epidemic

IF YOU ARE like most people, your day-to-day life is fraught with challenges. Trying to juggle all the responsibilities and obligations that come with life in our modern, fast-paced society can be mind-numbing. Worse yet, we've come to accept this as the status quo; stress and anxiety are just a part of life. We ignore the more serious short and long-term consequences that come from a life lived under constant pressure.

We live in a time when there are advancements in health being made every day, yet mood disorders are reaching pandemic levels across all age groups:

- **Adults**: 43.8 million (or 18.5 percent) of adult Americans suffer with mental illness per year.[1] Of these, 9.8 million (or 4.0 percent) deal with serious mental problems per year, which limits one or more main life activities.[2]
- **Youths**: 1 in 5 youths (ages 13–18 years) experience a severe mental episode during their life.[3]
- **Children**: 13.3 percent of children (ages 8–15) experience severe emotional/mental problems.[3]

Complicating matters is the number of different illnesses grouped under the heading of "mood disorder," many of which require unique forms of treatment:

- Schizophrenia (1.1 percent of adults)[4]
- Bipolar (2.6 percent of adults)[5]

- Anxiety (18.1 percent of adults)[6]
- Substance disorders (20.2 million adults); of these, 50.5 percent (10.2 million) also suffer with mental illness[7]

Against this, society as a whole is now fighting back, whether against their advancing years or poorer health, using nutraceuticals—natural, curative supplements that often times are less expensive than medications, both in terms of financial cost and the cost to one's long-term health. There is also a growing awareness of our environmental stressors (pollutants, insecticides, GMOs), driving people toward natural products and organically sourced foods.

Stress Plays a Big Part

Stress is a major contributing factor to many disease conditions, not the least of which include anxiety, depression, deviant behavior, chronic fatigue and bipolar disorder. Stress has become a steppingstone to the development of these disorders and many others, such as cardiovascular disease, chronic skin conditions and more.

Emotional and physical stress is the key obstacle that must be addressed to fully restore and preserve good health. If you are currently experiencing high levels of these stressors, there will need to be lifestyle changes and dietary adjustments made to bring you back to a healthy physical state.

To aid in this process, we have access to a wealth of natural medicine that can help bridge the gap between, or else augment the effects of certain medications. Sadly, the average person has at best only a vague understanding of what their body needs to remain not only healthy, but happy. Nutrients that boost your metabolism, immune system and energy levels; nutrients that reduce systemic inflammation; your body has requirements for its proper mental and physical function, which are particularly important for those looking to reverse the effects of their anxiety, depression, and chronic mood disorders.

The Growth of Natural Supplements Use

The last few decades have seen an explosive growth in the number of active natural health practitioners. This surge has been mirrored in parallel by a decline in the pharmaceutical industry, as more and more people seek alternatives to drugs. The lack of permanent results and unwanted side-effects has put this industry under public scrutiny, prompting many to look elsewhere for solutions—something which the pharmaceutical industry understandably wants to avoid, given that the sale of psychiatric drugs totals a staggering $80 billion profit per year.[8]

It is from a desire to set the record straight, and provide simple, straightforward guidance on how to care for your complete body health using supplements and nutraceuticals, that this book was created. And to start with, we will work from a very simple principle: if someone is experiencing declining health, there must be a reason. Likewise, if someone is experiencing a life without illness or negative symptoms, there must be a reason for that, too. Understanding what can be done to improve our health and reverse the course of our illness is the foundation of the protocols in this book.

This is a mystery that can be unraveled. For example, the average individual cannot avoid exposure to some form of environmental toxins, be it chemically laden foods or food devoid of needed nutrients. The answer to this problem is dietary supplements, which can replace or restore absent nutrients to correct long-term imbalances in the body.

In my personal and professional experience, I've seen two major scenarios that cause people to feel emotionally and physically burdened. One concerns a person's nutritional balance, in which the individual is missing key nutrients necessary for proper mental, hormonal and nerve balancing. The second is more common, and is a circumstance that many of us find ourselves stuck in: through the normal course of our life, we become overwhelmed by events outside our control which, coupled with ongoing fatigue, combines to stimulate negative thinking, leading to unhealthy life choices.

In other words, the first *physical* manifestations of mood imbalance and a lack of coping skills stem from a shortage of crucial nutrients required for proper body/brain functioning and signaling message transference. Natural therapeutics can help with this, connecting the broken links in the body's chain, regulating metabolism, rebuilding neurotransmitters, balancing hormone levels, and raising the immune system's ability to cope with outside toxins.

Understanding Depression

But the mental component of depression is a bit trickier. When you find yourself stuck in a quagmire of negative thinking, and everything in your life only serves to get you more and more trapped, eating healthier doesn't provide enough of a boost. To better understand what will be necessary to support your emotional and mental recovery process, we need to take a closer look at just what these disorders are.

The American Psychiatric Association (APA) describes it thusly in the Diagnostic and Statistical Manual of Mental Disorders 5th Edition:

"A mental disorder is a syndrome characterized by clinically significant disturbance in an individual's cognition, emotion regulation, or behavior that reflects a dysfunction in the psychological, biological, or developmental processes underlying mental functioning. Mental disorders are usually associated with significant distress or disability in social, occupational, or other important activities. An expectable or culturally approved response to a common stressor or loss, such as the death of a loved one, is not a mental disorder. Socially deviant behavior (e.g., political, religious, or sexual) and conflicts that are primarily between the individual and society are not mental disorders unless the deviance or conflict results from a dysfunction in the individual, as described above (APA, 2013, p. 20)."

Brain Nutrient Requirements

The brain, which represents 2 percent of our body weight, oversees a wide range of dietary nutrients. Our brain processes different fatty acids, as well as 20 amino acids and approximately 15 minerals and vitamins, in addition to carbohydrate assimilation and more.[9]

Now, with all these moving parts and specific requirements, imagine the effect on a young, developing brain when there is a *lack* of vital nutrition. Naturally, proper brain development and functionality would be affected. When a brain has not been properly supported nutritionally during its developmental stage, the person becomes more susceptible to cognitive and behavioral problems. There will be a decrease in brain cells and myelin production as well as a lower number of synapses; there may also be alterations in the neurotransmitter system such as in the release of chemical messenger neurotransmitters.

Neuronal communication is not possible without these messengers, and neurotransmitters must have adequate nutrition in order to be synthesized.[10] The brain cannot conduct its complicated metabolic operations without these messengers.

So, how do we feed our brain?

First, understand that when we say "feed our brain," we really mean "supply our brain." It's not just nutrients that the brain needs to carry out its duties: it also needs 20 percent of our body's oxygen, 25 percent of its total glucose intake, and 15 percent of our cardiac output. For the brain to survive, it requires 0.1 percent of our calories per minute in order to keep up with energy demands and survive.[11]

Quite the demand to fill. But making matters worse are issues with the quality of nutrient supply we have readily available to us. The brain cannot receive sufficient quantities of certain nutrients/fats when they are not typically part of the North American diet. Even when a person is really making an effort to eat better, nutritional shortages have already been caused by the nature of their purchased items.[12]

Our food's nutritional value has been diminished over time due to:

- Soil depletion of trace nutrients and vitamin/minerals due to modern day agricultural practices
- Food processing, refining and storage methods
- Pollution (environmental and household) increasing our nutrient requirements
- Absorption problems due to medications as well as tobacco, caffeine, alcohol, recreational drugs, and overconsumption of things like soda

There *are* supplements that exist to help shore up these shortages; however, most people have no knowledge of what nutrients are needed to perform all the thousands of functions and processes occurring daily throughout their body. Once a body has been placed into a nutritionally imbalanced state, all it takes is time for symptoms of lower functionality to manifest—often simultaneously.

A malnourished body guarantees a malnourished brain.[13] When certain compounds are unavailable to the brain, we see disruptions in our central nervous system and all neurochemistry in our brain. There are also micronutrients necessary for managing oxidative stress, which when coupled with other deficiencies can lead to psychiatric disorders.[14]

Brain Nutrient Depletion Affects Behavior

The brain requires a broad spectrum of minerals, vitamins, healthy fats and other nutrients to perform properly. So what happens when it *doesn't* function properly?

Whether the result is aggressive behavior or other cognitive dysfunction, we have seen a global increase in the rate of violent acts in the last 10–15 years. Even though these are multifaceted issues, studies show that nutritional interventions can have a positive effect on various subclinical behavioral episodes like those of aggression or other pathological violence involving impulsiveness and crime.[15] (More on the topic of aggressive behavior and brain psychopathology can be found in Chapter 2.)

In these and similar circumstances, more awareness of the underlying neurobiology and biochemical root of emotional and aggressive behavior can help improve on these issues by helping the suffering individuals involved.[15,16]

Next, we'll be reviewing problems related to psychiatric medications and violent behavior, along with where our society stands on antidepressant medications. Do they cause more harm than good?

CHAPTER 2

Psychiatric Medications

ANTIDEPRESSANT MEDICATIONS ARE the typically prescribed treatment for depression, as well as a host of other mood disorders such as anxiety, bipolar disorder, schizophrenia, post-traumatic stress disorder, obsessive-compulsive disorder, substance abuse, chronic pain conditions, and even eating disorders. In fact, reports released by the U.S. Centers for Disease Control and Prevention showed approximately 1 out of every 10 people over the age of 12 is currently taking antidepressant medication. From 2005–2008, antidepressants ranked as the third most common prescription medication consumed by people of all ages, especially people between the ages of 18 and 44. In other words, millions of people are taking and being affected by antidepressants each year.

Medication Unsafe for Teens

There has been a sudden increase in teenage patients suffering from depression and complications of drug therapy treatment. The following supportive study is just one example of how brain disruptive chemicals can worsen an already-delicate balance, producing life threatening side-effects.

New research analysis has determined that Paxil is unsafe for teens. The Restoring Study 329 (2015) involved 275 adolescents diagnosed with major depression. The participants were divided in two groups. One group took paroxetine (20-40 mg) and imipramine (200-300 mg) while the second was placebo.

The first group taking the medications was not clinically or statistically different from the placebo group, for primary or secondary efficacy result. However, there were serious side effects such as suicidal tendencies. During

7

the double-blind treatment, 11 subjects, in the Paxil group engaged in suicidal acts, compared to 1 person in the placebo group.[1]

Due to the rise of depressive disorders ending in suicide and the incidence of deaths coinciding with aggressive behavior, the need for another approach is clear.

Granted, suicide is associated with the more severe types of depression like schizophrenia and bipolar disorder (*and* their medications). But by taking an integrative approach to suicidality, we present at-risk patients with the best opportunity for recovery. We have strong evidence showing how basic biochemical abnormalities and environmental issues affect the structure and functioning of our brains. The brain is also involved in the escalation of aggressive and violent behavior (discussed further on in this chapter).

The application of nutritional supplementation with other complementary interventions will help lessen risk factors of suicide while addressing the underlying biochemical individuality of a patient.[2]

Effects of Antidepressants on Aging Population

On the other end of the spectrum, antidepressants also have many negative effects on our aging population. There has been a great deal of research conducted on the ill effects of antidepressants and elderly patients, and there exist strong conclusions surrounding this age group.

Over long periods of time, the side effects of antidepressant medications can be considerable, leading to:[3,4]

- Cognitive decline
- Dementia/Alzheimer's disease
- Stroke
- Cardiovascular problems
- Gastrointestinal problems
- Death
- Hyponatremia (low sodium in blood plasma)
  - o Headaches
  - o Nausea
  - o Muscle cramps
  - o Lethargy
  - o Disorientation

- Severe cases of Hyponatremia could result in:
  - o Coma
  - o Seizures
  - o Respiratory arrest
  - o Death

Do Antidepressants Do More Harm than Good?

The hope is that medications treating mood disorders are safe and effective. However, recent scientific research is beginning to show ways in which antidepressant drugs may be more harmful than helpful—or reliable. The issues underlying the over-prescription of antidepressants is such that we find ourselves facing a serious health problem, one which may also have legal and ethical ramifications.

Let's first take a brief look at how most antidepressant medications work. The majority of antidepressants are formulated to alter our body's systems that regulate **serotonin**, which functions as a neurotransmitter in our brain. Serotonin is also found throughout the rest of our body, regulating the progression of neuronal cell growth and death, aiding in our digestion, muscle and bowel contractions, as well as affecting mood, sleep, libido/reproduction, blood clotting, and memory and learning. (We'll be discussing the role of serotonin in our body in greater detail in Chapter 3.)

Selective serotonin reuptake inhibitors (SSRIs), which comprise the majority of prescription antidepressants, are programmed to bind to a **serotonin transporter**, a molecule that regulates serotonin levels. Most antidepressant medications work the same way: when these drugs connect with the serotonin transporter, they prevent the neurons from reabsorbing serotonin, creating a build-up of serotonin on the outer surface of the neurons. By increasing serotonin concentration on the neurons, we create an imbalance of serotonin in the brain. The brain will eventually push back against these drugs by effecting a number of biological changes to restore the serotonin balance outside of the brain neurons. This in turn produces a limited duration of symptom benefit, due to the increase in mood regulating serotonin activity.

What Else is Impacted by SSRI Medications?

However, a problem presents itself that may not be obvious: because serotonin is found in many major sites in our body, the use of antidepressants to artificially inflate serotonin's concentrations produces harmful effects on important body functions and processes that are regulated by serotonin.

Specifically, you can expect to see adverse side effects like abnormal bleeding, digestion problems and sexual dysfunction. While you (and your doctor) may only be interested in how these drugs affect your mood, you need to realize that many of these side effects will further enhance depression and affect future health.

For example, say you are a young, single male with aspirations of interpersonal relationships, only to realize that a very important aspect of a healthy lifestyle (sexual activity) is no longer functioning normally. Do you think this scenario would heal a depressive state? Or would it create frustration and hopelessness, further supporting a mood disorder?[5]

This is why we can only say that antidepressants are moderately effective, and should not constitute a permanent, or even a long-term, treatment plan. Even though some patients report a substantial benefit while taking SSRIs, their benefits are due to the brain pushing back, as we described earlier. This means their positive benefit is limited and short-lived, by its very nature. Medical professionals continue to debate the degree of benefit antidepressants provide; however, reports consistently show only modest effects.[6]

Does a placebo work as well?

In evaluating the benefits experienced by patients taking antidepressants, and those taking a placebo, there were not any major differences between the two—with the exception that a placebo, or sugar pill, lacks the harmful chemical properties of antidepressants. They even demonstrated similar benefits in terms of timeline: both antidepressant medications and placebos were found to deliver the highest degree of symptom relief at roughly the same time. While antidepressants were found to deliver a higher degree of symptom relief, this difference was only marginal.[7,8]

It's all because of that "push back" brain effect: over subsequent months of treatment, symptoms of depression usually return, typically reaching a full scale relapse. Physicians then prescribe an increase of dosage, or another, more potent medication. It almost seems as though doctors are not properly taking into account the consequences of the brain pushing against the drugs (to rebalance itself), resulting in the patient's return of symptoms.

There is a reason for the surge of depressive symptoms seen following someone going off their antidepressant medications. This can be thought of as a build-up in pressure, similar to the action of a spring being compressed and then released. The symptoms are held in place for a time, while the medication is being taken—but when the SSRI is no longer present, there is a surge of returning symptoms as the spring is released.

By comparison, the risk of symptom relapse for those taking a placebo at 3 months was approximately 21 percent, while the relapse risk of SSRI medications was doubled, at 43 percent. Additionally, the 3-month relapse risk was much higher when stronger antidepressant drugs had been taken.[9,10,11]

Of course, there's more at risk when using antidepressants than their diminishing returns. The following are some of the additional risks incurred by the use (or misuse) of mood disorder medications.

Neuronal Damage and Death

Antidepressants cause structural damage to neurons, resulting in **neuronal death**, a condition similar to what is seen in the brains of Parkinson's patients. This may be one reason why some patients develop symptoms of Parkinsonian dementia when taking antidepressants.[12,13,14]

Brain Impairment

Let's not forget that neurons are a main feature of proper brain function; therefore, when we have neurons being destroyed by antidepressants, it is to be expected that we would see negative effects on our cognition.

Brain impairment due to antidepressant usage is further supported by animal studies, including rodent studies wherein prolonged usage of antidepressants was found to impair their ability to learn and perform a variety of tasks. For older women, owning to prolonged antidepressant use, research shows a 70 percent increased risk of dementia and mild cognitive impairment.[15]

Inflammation and Depression
You may be wondering: how can depression be related to inflammation? What would be examples of sources of this type of inflammation? The answer is that our immune system is directly involved with initiating our inflammation response; therefore, vitamin D deficiency, allergies, stress, gut dysbiosis, environmental chemicals and pollution, the standard American diet, key nutrient deficiencies such as B vitamins, vitamins, minerals, essential fatty acids and amino acids, inadequate sleep and others all contribute to an inflammation response—as well as worsen depression symptoms.

Behavioral Complications of Antidepressants

So far, we've discussed the inherent medical limitations of antidepressants, as well as their negative effects on the body and harmful interactions with other drugs. However, the widespread use of antidepressants presents additional, behavioral issues; and as depression is at once a physical and mental disorder, these additional dangers should be explored and understood.

Aggressive Behavior
The term "aggressive behavior" covers a range of action patterns, from verbal abuse to deadly physical violence.[16]

Characterized as a mental disorder, aggressive behavior is broken down into the following categories:
- Post-traumatic stress disorder (PTSD)
- Intermittent explosive disorder
- Irritable aggression
- Depression-linked aggression
- Increased autonomic arousal (sudden and uncontrolled reactive aggression)

Societies worldwide are dealing with an alarming death rate due to violent behavior. Of these, domestic violence and other violent acts are steadily on the rise, in turn warranting more education and stricter regulations of law enforcement.[17]

School Shootings and Antidepressants

Unwanted or inappropriate behaviors fueled by drug side effects and a lack of proper brain/body nutrition has developed into a major societal problem. Aggressive and violent behavior has escalated to the point that traumatic events involving school shootings have become more commonplace than ever before.

Research supports the involvement of antidepressant medications in the prevalence of these incidences, due either to the medications these individuals are taking, or else weaning off. Few have begun to address this area of concern, focusing instead on the related issue of gun control.[18] For more collaborative information on this topic, review the section on blood and urine tests in Chapter 3.

Aggression and Brain Psychopathology

The causes of aggressive and violent behavior typically involve the brain's biology and biochemical structure. We are aware of specific neurotransmitters that are implicated with aggression, cognition and other psychiatric disorders,[19,20] but what of the contributing factors that set up a person to manifest these inappropriate behaviors?

For example, early indicators of childhood ADHD, especially when combined with an unhealthy family environment and learning difficulties, have often resulted in delinquent behavior during adolescent years. As of 2016, 30.8 percent of criminal offenders possessed both ADHD and behavior disorders. Another problem to deal with is the prevalence of substance abuse and the development of addictions, all of which enhance abusive and violent behavior.[21]

As a practitioner who often treats conditions of ADHD and autism, the process isn't dissimilar to treating cognitive imbalance/deficiency in adults. The brain and the endocrine system require special attention, as a rule, and the body as a whole must be nutritionally supported. But the focus in these instances is mainly on supporting neurotransmitters, key glands (thyroid, adrenals, hypothalamus, and pituitary), maintaining amino acid balance and reducing brain inflammation, primarily through antioxidants.

While taking into account social and biochemical factors, a continued lack of proper nutrient support creates higher vulnerability, especially during chronic stress events. During such circumstances (such as emotional outbursts), the body requires vast amounts of nutrients to cope with the increased energy requirements of our body. Coupled with prolonged stress and a lack of quality nutrition, all *negative* aspects of emotional and general health will continue to worsen.

Behavioral Issues and Malnutrition

Numerous studies have shown specific dietary absences to be associated with a predisposition towards violence, crime and antisocial conduct. This relationship was shown to exist between maladaptive behaviors and the following: chemical additives, food sensitivities and intolerances, sugar consumption, lack of fatty acids, low mineral/vitamin intake along with the development of hypoglycemia.[22]

Further studies confirm the benefits of better-quality nutrition in adults with mood disorders and deviant behavior. Improved mental health in conjunction with increased nutrient intake resulted in studies showing a need for nutrient digestion and psychiatric performance.[23,24]

We have reviewed many complications involving antidepressant and psych medications, including their physical impact on our body systems and their negative emotional and behavioral side effects, as well as their extended usage problems. Overall, the number of side effects associated with SSRIs is extensive—and still growing. In the following chapter, we will go into more depth on the role serotonin plays in our body, as well as the related issue of tryptophan depletion. Take careful notice of how specific nutrients are needed to support the body, especially when major imbalances occur causing unnatural behavior.

CHAPTER 3

Serotonin and Tryptophan

OUR PHYSICAL BODY will not feel healthy while we have an unhealthy mind. Likewise, our mental health deteriorates when we have nutrient deficiencies and an imbalance of certain chemicals. Mind-body health, therefore, rests on maintaining a certain balance, one which is all too often thrown off by the stresses of modern life and the holes in our modern diet and nutritionally depleted food supply.

One such imbalance occurs when levels of the neurotransmitter **serotonin** become deficient. Serotonin assists in our mood regulation; therefore, when our brain is deficient in this chemical symptoms of depression, anxiety, and even insomnia can present themselves. The use of SSRIs and other antidepressant medications can temporarily inflate our serotonin levels as the body rebounds, working in overdrive to achieve a balance, but the short-term benefits and long-term ill effects of these medications discourage their repeated use.

So, to help steer away from antidepressant medications, we need to find more natural solutions to boost and maintain serotonin levels. But first, we need to discuss in a bit more detail exactly what serotonin is, and how it works in our bodies.

Serotonin in Our Body

Serotonin is a neurotransmitter derived from the essential amino acid **tryptophan** (chemical name, 5-Hydroxytryptamine or 5-HT).[1]

Serotonin is produced in our gastrointestinal tract and brain, and is also found in our central nervous system and blood platelets.[2] A brief list of serotonin's many functions in our body include influencing our brain cells in ways related to mood, as well as regulating libido and sexual function, memory, learning, sleep, appetite, body temperature and even certain social behaviors. It also affects the performance of our cardiovascular system and muscles, and influences a number of aspects in the endocrine system.[3]

Serotonin Deficiency

There are a number of substances that contribute to permanently damaging the nerves cells that produce serotonin and other neurotransmitters. Primary offenders include heavy metals, pesticides, medication use and certain prescription drugs; as well, a lack of sunlight can decrease serotonin levels.[4]

Integrative Psychiatry reports a variety of body and psychological symptoms attributed to low serotonin levels,[5] including:

- Depression
- Anxiety
- Eating disorders
- Panic attacks
- Low self-esteem
- OCD (Obsessive Compulsive Disorder)
- Negative thoughts
- Insomnia
- Alcohol abuse
- Chronic pain
- Obesity
- Fibromyalgia
- Migraines
- IBS (Irritable Bowel Syndrome)
- PMS (Premenstrual Syndrome)

Testing for Serotonin Levels

When testing for serotonin levels in the body, typically a blood and/or urine test will be performed. Based on the results on these tests, the individual will be evaluated against five different forms of clinical depression recognized by medical professionals. The study which identified these five types, led by William J. Walsh, Ph.D., (president of the Walsh Research Institute), saw Dr. Walsh and his team review about 300,000 blood and urine test results (in addition to 200,000 medical history facts) from roughly 2,800 patients that had been diagnosed with depression. They concluded that five major depression types were characterized in about 95 percent of the patients.[6]

From the results of this test, Dr. Walsh and his team determined that three forms of depression *were not* due to fluctuating serotonin levels, further emphasizing the importance of testing serotonin levels of patients with depression symptoms to help rule out potential causes. (However, most psychiatrists still believe all depression cases to be caused by low serotonin levels; this is why their go-to treatment involves serotonin re-uptake inhibitors (SSRIs).)[7]

Dr. Walsh goes on to say, "We are not the first to suggest that there may be other causes of depression, but we might be the first to identify the other forms of depression, and the first to suggest blood testing to guide the treatment approach."

In brief, here are the five types of depression as determined by Walsh and his team:

Undermethylated depression. This form of depression was found in 38 percent of the study subjects. Dr. Walsh states, "It's not serotonin deficiency, but an inability to keep serotonin in the synapse long enough. Most of these patients report excellent response to SSRI antidepressants, although they may experience nasty side effects."

Pyrrole depression. This type of depression was noted in 17 percent of the patients, who expressed that they felt helped by the antidepressants (SSRIs). These participants displayed high levels of oxidative stress with low production of serotonin.

Copper overload. In this case, found in 15 percent of patients in the study (mostly women), individuals could not metabolize heavy metals, including estrogen. The patients also reported indifference to the SSRIs medications—neither positive nor negative results. Their high copper levels were normalized through natural nutritional therapy.

Dr. Walsh further comments, "For them, it's not a serotonin issue, but extreme blood and brain levels of copper that result in dopamine deficiency and norepinephrine overload; this may be the primary cause of postpartum depression."

Low-folate depression. This group comprised 20 percent of the study and reported that SSRIs made their symptoms worse. It was only with the addition of folic acid and B12 supplements that their negative symptoms were reduced. Dr. Walsh went on to say, after evaluating fifty school shootings over the past fifty years, that these violent offenders most likely had problems with SSRIs; these drugs can cause homicidal and suicidal thought patterns in certain cases. (More information on why low folate levels can lead to depression is found in Chapter 11.)

Toxic depression. Toxicity from metals (in this case, normally lead poisoning) accounts for 5 percent of the patient study. On a positive note, the removal of lead from paint and gasoline has lowered this toxic metal problem somewhat.

While Dr. Walsh has stated his goal is to train and educate doctors in this new form of evaluation and testing, some doctors have expressed doubts, saying that there are too few researchers advancing this area of study. A psychiatrist operating out of Boston, David Brendel M.D., Ph.D., applauded the program, saying it was a "significant advance" in using medical tests to diagnose forms of depression. He went on to say, however: "I don't see adequate evidence that these [or other] researchers are anywhere near accomplishing this," arguing the medical community is "entirely unable" to competently diagnose depression using medical tests, due to its many social and neurophysiological causes.[8]

Tryptophan Depletion and Serotonin

Tryptophan depletion is a widely used study model to help determine if there are any abnormalities in the serotonin function of depressed patients. A key reason for this research is to help improve the accuracy of current diagnostic categories of depression, and to better understand the nerve/brain pathology.[9]

By assessing the neurobiology of depressive disorders in an effort to improve treatment outcomes, doctors will examine the prefrontal and limbic areas of the brain, with particular emphasis on the hippocampus, looking for any structural or functional changes of the nervous system in these brain areas.[10]

The effects of **acute tryptophan depletion (ATD)** on cognitive function and mood have also been investigated in separate studies looking to test individual vulnerability. Those with a family history of depression (while ATD remained in effect) did experience lower moods; even those subjects without mood disorder predisposition saw lower moods while undergoing this study. Memory impairment was noted in all study participants while under the influence of acute tryptophan depletion. This model of study can hopefully be used to assess patient susceptibility towards serotonin neurobiology.[11]

Supplements that Increase Serotonin Levels

While more detailed information on healthful supplements to help reverse depression and support whole body health can be found in subsequent chapters, the following are particularly helpful for managing serotonin levels and improving tryptophan production.

L-Tryptophan
L-Tryptophan is an essential amino acid required by our body to manufacture serotonin. 5-HTP is made from tryptophan; in other words, our bodies make 5-hydroxy tryptophan (5-HTP) from tryptophan, and then convert it into serotonin.[12]

SAMe
SAMe (s-adenosyl methionine) is new to the North American market, having been available since 1999; however, it has been studied for decades worldwide, even being approved in Germany, Italy, Russia and Spain as a prescription drug. In excess of one million Europeans have used SAMe for depression and for arthritic pain relief.[12]

Omega-3 Fatty Acids
Omega-3 fatty acids are derived from fish oil, flaxseed, and evening primrose oil (among other sources) and help kickstart and boost neurotransmitter signals between the synapses in the brain, resulting in improved serotonin function in those areas.[13]

St. John's Wort
Similar to Omega-3 Fatty acids, St. John's Wort stimulates the signals in our nerve endings and synapses, helping them to work more efficiently. Overall, the flow of serotonin in the brain circulates more effortlessly when

using St. John's wort, helping to regulate moods while also improving mental focus.[14]

Vitamin D

Vitamin D deficiency has a strong association with depression and anxiety, in addition to many other disorders. In this instance, vitamin D is needed to help convert tryptophan into serotonin.[15] Recently, this vitamin is showing to be deficient in most people, largely due to lack of sun exposure.

Magnesium

Magnesium is one of the most influential elements in our bodies, and its benefits extend to treating the major types of depression. It assists in serotonin balance, along with its many other duties including boosting nervous system function.[16]

Zinc

Zinc works closely with magnesium throughout our body and enhances brain function by supporting the signals between nerve endings in the brain. Because zinc can increase serotonin uptake in certain parts of the brain, it can also help increase serotonin levels and improve moods.[17]

Vitamin B

B vitamins are very supportive when combined with other supplements to increase serotonin levels. Specifically, Vitamin B6 is required to convert tryptophan into serotonin, while B12 and B9 must be present for SAMe to be utilized by the brain.[18]

L-Theanine

L-Theanine is an amino acid derived from green tea that has been shown to increase serotonin levels while also offering support against the harmful effects of stress. Additionally, it provides a calming effect in some individuals.[19]

Curcumin

Curcumin offers a variety of benefits and is a recent addition to this list, having been now shown to increase serotonin and dopamine levels. The absorption and bioavailability of curcumin is this supplement's only drawback, so be sure to look for products that have greatly decreased particle size in order to boost its absorption rate.[20]

Now that we have a better understanding of the various causes of depression—be it low serotonin levels or other nutrient deficiencies—it becomes easier to see why traditional antidepressants can only serve as an imprecise stopgap measure. It is not unlike a drug addict, always chasing a better or more effective high; only here, we have the added downside of a "crash" leading to an even deeper, more entrenched form of depression.

In the next chapter, we'll be exploring the disorder of depression in greater detail, examining its symptoms, warning signs, and treatment options available for those looking for more than the quick fix the traditional medicinal route provides.

CHAPTER 4

Types of Depression

D EPRESSIVE DISORDERS VARY in severity of symptoms, so it's important to be clear on what "type" of depression we mean when beginning a discussion. The information in this section will focus on the 'lighter side' of depression—individuals who suffer from depression, but can still handle their day-to-day routines—to those with mood disorders that interfere with most aspects of their life, whether due to anxiety, major depression disorder or bipolar disorder.

Hidden Symptoms of Depression and Anxiety

The symptoms of depression can be very noticeable, but this is not always the case: there are individuals who have mastered 'the art of disguise', hiding their true feelings from even those closest to them. Often times, these individuals believe the way they feel is normal, or choose not to speak out for fear of embarrassment or judgment. These issues are so common-place and critical to any discussion of depressive disorders that we must discuss them in greater detail before proceeding on.

Perfectly Hidden Depression
Do you think you have depression? Do you want help? Are you pretending that you are fine and your ill feelings are simply what you consider to be normal?

These are the sorts of self-evaluating questions that standard depression tests will ask to help individuals determine if they should pursue treatment for their negative feelings. Yet there are a surprising number of categories that the symptoms of depression fall under, and taking a depression test does not always give an accurate account of someone's current mental state.

(For instance, self-scoring depression tests will only show what a person wants someone to see.)

There are many people who suffer with moderate forms of depression in silence, assuming the way they feel and function to be normal.[1,2] Persons of this description are far more likely to fall under the radar, having learned to blend in while putting up with their symptoms. These individuals are in denial, and are unable or unwilling to let someone see their real depression test scores, for example—which means they are not seeking help.

This group falls under a category called **Perfectly Hidden Depression (PHD)**.[3]

Compared to the more well-known labels for mood disorders, these individuals often go unnoticed, leading to devastating outcomes, especially if the individual is contemplating taking their life. Sadly, no one has any idea of their personal struggle, and therefore cannot offer any assistance.

It may help to look at some of the known characteristics of PHD, which may provide a clue as to who is silently calling for help.[4]

Denial. As mentioned earlier, individuals with PHD do not want to believe they are depressed, leading them to disguise their state of mind. When asked questions about how they feel, they will typically not answer honestly.

Emotionally detached. Unlike most people with depressive disorders, PHD persons suffer in silence. They like to unravel their problems on an analytical level, in their own minds. They do their best to avoid angry outbursts, as well as numbing their feelings of sadness or disappointments, 'choosing' to smile their way through life. Their need for control is always evident.

Compartmentalized feelings. Persons with PHD develop above-average skills at compartmentalizing their past or present hurts or painful feelings. We all have this capability—it's one of our coping mechanisms as humans—however, people with PHD tend to over-rationalize bad life experiences, feeling that because others have gone through much worse, they have no right to feel sad or complain. They may even suppress happy feelings, believing it not to be the time to express themselves.

Even though people with PHD work very hard at hiding their feelings, there *are* indicators, albeit ones that may go unnoticed. Take note of infrequent outbursts of anger or what would seem like abnormal behavior, like uncommon irritability. Men are more inclined to express their depression in this way than women.

Lack of disclosure. It can be very traumatic for people with PHD, who bottle everything up, to share their past hurtful events—even with those close to them who are aware of such events. A major problem for everyone, not just PHD persons, is constant underlying negative thought processes, which in their case can lead to suicidal thoughts. A person with PHD will attempt to hide an overwhelming problem such as suicidal tendencies, fearing no one would believe them, since their outward expression is one of 'all is well'.

Empathy. Someone with PHD can show sincere concern for others and may even be a great care provider, as by helping others they ward off any signs that they themselves may need assistance or may be feeling over-whelmed.[5]

Camouflage. People with PHD tend to deflect attention away from themselves, having developed various coping mechanisms to do so. For example, they will appear to be happy, even extroverted at times; or else they will demonstrate the reverse, standing back in a crowd so as not to draw any attention. They often maintain good jobs and put other's needs before their own, while being loving and reliable. When an individual appears to be happy and balanced, it can prove difficult for them to get the help they need—and to get an accurate diagnosis of their imbalance.[5]

Abnormal eating habits. This area is not clear-cut, as today we see widespread instances of imbalanced diets, but some mood disorders can be contributed to by gut dysbiosis or by very poor diets creating mood swings and chronic fatigue.[6]

Likewise, diets high in sugar and chemicals directly impact the addictive center of our brains. The more you eat or drink, the more you will desire those additives; this is why sugar is associated with depressive moods and weight gain. Carbohydrates from white flour, as well as bad fats, will further enhance this scenario. If you notice a real change in someone's eating habits, open a discussion with them and note the changes you've observed, as a precursor to providing them any help or support they need.

Gut bacteria. A body whose digestive system is overrun with yeast, fungus and other pathogens automatically equates to a less-than-optimally functioning immune system. Bipolar disorder, schizophrenia and other mood disorders have been associated with abnormal amounts of *candida Albicans* (a yeast-like fungus) in the brain tissue.[7,8]

A leaky gut will result in lower thyroid function due to gluten creating an autoimmune response. Gluten and thyroid tissue present an almost identical matrix to the body, meaning the immune system cannot differentiate between the two and attacks the thyroid gland whenever gluten is ingested. As the thyroid gland is directly tied to various neurotransmitters that create good moods and energy, all of which will be lower functioning due to hypothyroidism, an unhealthy gut can create the symptoms of a mood disorder.[6]

Abnormal personal goals. While doing your best is an admirable quality, a person with PHD may take things to an unreasonable level. This will most often have to do with their job or a particular interest or hobby.[4,5] Their constant attempts at perfectionism can be a telltale sign. Look for those who berate themselves unnecessarily when their personal expectations are not met. Unfortunately, most will usually remain silent, keeping their perceived inadequacies to themselves.

Anxiety. Many mental health issues have a component of anxiety; however, in the instance of people with PHD, they will attempt to deal with their anxiety in a strictly controlled fashion. It is not uncommon for these individuals to either seek escape from or control of their anxiety by means of being obsessive compulsive, involving an eating disorder and/or the use of alcohol or psychiatric medications.[4,5]

Control. This may be difficult to diagnose accurately, as there are many personality types who like to have things their own way; those who prefer to lead rather than follow, someone who wants to be in control. However, there are a few signs that may point to an individual suffering with PHD, such as obsessing about every little detail—especially when whatever they are doing *should* be stress-free. You may notice they have a hard time relaxing and settling down to enjoy the moment or appreciating what they have just accomplished.[4,5] The need for control shows itself in the person's unnecessary worry over 'what if's' that might occur to disrupt their controlled environment.

Anxiety Disorders

The term "anxiety disorder" is somewhat broad and non-descriptive, as there are a host of symptomatologies that fall under this heading. The term anxiety can be defined as "a perceived threatening or frightening event response"—something which, under warranted circumstances, is a normal body response to anticipated danger. It is when we see abnormal, repetitive fear responses to events that would not normally elicit these reactions by most people that we find cause for concern.

There are several types of common anxiety disorders, all of which fall under the heading of generalized anxiety disorder (GAD), a catch-all term first introduced to the medical world in the Diagnostic and Statistical Manual of Mental Disorders, Third Edition (or DSM-III). Examples include obsessive compulsive disorder (OCD), panic disorder (PD), phobias, social anxiety disorder, and post-traumatic stress disorder, among others.[9]

While accurate estimates are hard to obtain, the National Institute of Mental Health reports that 19 million Americans (approximately 13 percent) have anxiety disorders, most commonly in ages ranging between 18–54 years.[10] The question has also been raised as to whether GAD is actually a separate condition, or if its symptoms should be considered as part of the progression of a depressive mood disorder.[11]

Most Widely Used Drugs for Anxiety

Serotonin reuptake inhibitors (specifically fluoxetine and fluvoxamine) were introduced in the 1980s for the treatment of depression, and quickly became one of the most frequently prescribed medications in the world. Generally referred to as the SSRIs, the function (and negative impact) of these medications has been discussed in the previous chapter; however, they have also seen wide use in the treatment of anxiety in both pediatric and adult patients[12,13,14,15]

However, there are unique shortcomings when considering these medications for the treatment of acute anxiety—namely their delayed treatment response. The lag time of these medications make them a poor choice for individuals who experience episodes of extreme anxiety; in addition, certain side effects are another cause for concern, including weight gain, sexual dysfunction, agitation and insomnia.[13,16,17] Another drawback is the number of negative drug interactions found with certain SSRIs; for patients who are on several other medications, the introduction of anxiety medication can do more harm than good.[18]

So, what is the solution? Given that the primary medical response is lacking, addressing these shortcomings becomes a primary focal point for holistic treatment of anxiety. Of course, even suggesting the use of holistic treatment methods is a major hurdle for some, since most people have only experienced treatment protocols involving medication. Because of this lack of experience and knowledge of alternate solutions, fear, nervousness, and doubt are common reactions upon first suggesting the replacement of problematic drugs. Yet even drugs that seem tolerable will still have long-term efficacy problems or other drug interactions problems[18], plus other physical side effects.[13]

For instance, this family of drugs has a tendency to result in brain fog and dementia the longer one remains on certain types of medications. Known brain disrupters that lead to dementia include medications prescribed for depression and sleep, with the next most common being antihistamines for allergies and skin issues.

Drug Addiction Problems

When prescribing medications for the treatment of anxiety, it can be difficult for the doctor/clinician to pinpoint patient symptoms that may be indicative of future problems with certain medications, such as benzodiazepines, and abuse potential.[19] Identifying a potential addict is not always an easy task, yet the medical establishment is still faced with the possible issues of drug dependency and medical safety when developing a prescription treatment plan.

For patients who exhibit great difficulty in stopping their drug, suggesting psychological and physical drug dependence, this is often indicative of a reemergence of their initial symptoms of depression and phobias. As well, there appears to be a relationship between other substance addictions, like alcohol or smoking, and anxiety disorders.[20-27] For patients who *do* have a history of substance abuse, the current conventional recommendation is to not prescribe benzodiazepines, as these patients have an increased risk of developing a dependence on this class of drugs.[14]

Major Depressive Disorder and Bipolar

Major depressive disorder (MDD) describes a collection of symptoms including fatigue, fluctuation in weight or appetite, depressive moods, slowing of mental activity for movement and things that once were pleasurable no longer holding interest.[28] When one thinks of depression, this is typically the disorder that comes to mind.

Bipolar disorder, previously called manic depression, has more pronounced symptoms than major depressive disorder. A person with bipolar will experience extreme mood swings, longer periods of depression, racing thoughts, hyperactivity, a feeling of invincibility and being larger-than-life, as well as grandiose delusions.[29] The latter of which, described as a **manic episode,** can cause significant distress to one's family environment and eventually impairs one's work and social life.[30] Anyone who has lived with a bipolar patient can most likely attest to their prolonged agitated states, in which they act obsessed about something that they think has taken place but may not have. Trying to reason with them only brings out angry outbursts, or else they may have periods (lasting several days) of simmering emotions of anger, followed by bursts of rage.[31]

Similarly, it is possible for a person with MDD to experience a depressive episode and not be bipolar. The symptoms are different, albeit similar in some surface aspects; a major depressive episode would involve symptoms that last two weeks or longer, as already described, in addition to feelings of hopelessness, sadness, sleep problems and suicidal thoughts.[32]

Major depressive disorder, if left untreated and unresolved, can lead to bipolar. Bipolar involving depressive episodes may progress to violence, substance abuse and even suicide.[33] It is therefore essential that individuals struggling with these issues receive proper support and treatment. While it may be possible for MDD to go away on its own without treatment, it is far more likely that symptoms will worsen before they improve. This is a chronic condition, one where a person may experience periods of improvement but also low periods of depression.[34]

Is it Bipolar or Depression?

Not surprisingly, many people who are diagnosed with major depression may also be bipolar, since they both experience many of the same symptoms—with the exception of mania. Some patients who have been diagnosed with clinical depression by their doctors actually have bipolar disorder and have been inaccurately diagnosed. It all hinges on the symptoms presenting at the time when the doctors make their evaluation.

There is, however, a major hurdle when depression *becomes part of* bipolar. Bipolar disorders like schizophrenia can be devastating, both to the family and the individual. Major mood disorders can be debilitating to the point of a person not being able to function normally. Normal routines like showering or getting out of bed become challenging, as does going to work or pursuing activities that were once enjoyed. And then there are the unwanted thoughts, including those of suicide. All in all, it paints a very bleak picture for all concerned.

Roger S. McIntyre, MD, is an associate professor of psychiatry and pharmacology at the University of Toronto, and head of the Mood Disorders Psychopharmacology Unit at the University Health Network in Toronto. He comments on major depression and bipolar disorders *and* the problems of antidepressant usage: "You look at the functional outcomes, such as the ability to work, family life, being an active participant in society—this is largely driven by depressive, rather than manic, symptoms." Dr. McIntyre continues, "Bipolar depression looks very similar to major depression, with no distinct features. That being said, people with bipolar depression more often complain of symptoms that are atypical for unipolar depression, including increased eating, sleeping, and profound reduction in energy. Moreover, people with bipolar depression also frequently complain of seasonal worsening and 'therapeutic misadventures' with antidepressants—that is, the depression gets worse with antidepressant therapy."[35]

Alternative Treatment of Depression

At first glance, you may not find a lot of specific alternative remedies for manic behavior, yet there are several choices that can be taken individually or combined for greater effect when needed. But more than that is the need for combined physical and mental support provided by propping up key systems and mental pathways, support that medications cannot provide.

Healing is achieved by balancing and supporting areas that are weak and not functioning normally. By providing these missing links and temporary calming elements, unpredictable symptoms are reduced while positive energy and good feelings resurface. This healing method also diminishes drug withdrawals, all the while paving the way for a successful recovery.

When starting the healing process for serious mood disorders, begin with the 'Initial Protocol' provided in Chapter 9, and review the schizophrenia case history on page 35 for many other helpful suggestions in accomplishing the reversal process.

In the next chapter, we'll continue to pursue our discussion of the dangers of bipolar disorder by delving deeper into the illness known as schizophrenia. While the topic of this discussion is limited to this disorder, the information provided is also very helpful for anyone looking for a better way to treat this disease and other life-changing mood disorders. In particular, the extensive case history of a schizophrenia patient—with full details of their road to recovery—provides a sample roadmap for treatment of mood disorders without the use of potentially harmful medications.

CHAPTER 5

Schizophrenia

SCHIZOPHRENIA IS A severe and chronic form of debilitating mental illness which, while not as common as other mental disorders, can completely alter a person's current and future life direction. Persons suffering with this condition will appear to have lost touch with reality; it affects how they feel, how they process their surroundings, and how they conduct themselves.

As of 2014, this severe neurological brain illness was found to affect 1.1 percent of the U.S. population (approximately 2.6 million adults, age 18 or older).[1] The disease typically begins between the ages of 15 and 25 for men, while women seem to become afflicted much later (after the age of 30). Like most illnesses, the earlier a person is diagnosed and treated, the better their chances of full recovery—especially when treated holistically.[2,3]

Risk Factors for Schizophrenia

Recently, scientists have made an unexpected discovery linking schizophrenia to genes involved in the normal course of development. When combined with certain environmental exposures, or problems during pregnancy and malnutrition before birth, or childhood circumstances, these genes can begin to function improperly, potentially leading to the development of schizophrenia later in life. Researchers have identified specific genes, like DISC1, Dysbindin, Neuregulin and G72 genes; however, there may be many more genes involved in this neurological disorder.[4]

In addition to faulty genes, we cannot overlook our brain chemistry and structure. Disturbances in our brain's chemical reactions (interference with neurotransmitter activity) results in our brain cells' inability to communicate with one another. This creates imbalances, particularly when the disruption involves dopamine, glutamate, or serotonin and tryptophan levels, among other substances.

Symptoms and Signs

When diagnosing schizophrenia, patients will generally fall into one of three categories: positive, negative and cognitive.

Positive Symptoms of Schizophrenia

Positive symptoms of schizophrenia describe psychotic behaviors not normally seen in a healthy patient, such as losing touch with certain aspects of reality.

The following are examples of positive symptoms:

- Hallucinations
- Delusions
- Thought disorders (abnormal or dysfunctional thoughts)
- Movement disorders (nervous, uneasy or slow body movements)

Negative Symptoms of Schizophrenia

Negative symptoms are considered to be those that disrupt usual behaviors and emotions.

Some examples include:

- Lack of expression in facial or voice tone (flat affect)
- Lack of daily pleasure and interest in everyday life (apathy)
- Focus problems; difficulty starting an activity and sticking with it
- Less verbal; becoming less self-expressive and quieter

Cognitive Symptoms of Schizophrenia
Cognitive symptoms will vary from patient to patient, and may be subtle or more severe.

Indicators include:

- Problems with decision-making and execution

- Difficulties with paying attention and concentrating on tasks
- Slow mental processing
- Difficulty retaining what was just learned *and* applying the information

Paranoid Schizophrenia

Paranoia is a distinguishing symptom of this illness, but it can be very unpredictable as to when it shows up, and how. As symptoms become more pronounced, the patient's life will change dramatically, as will those of their caregivers. It becomes difficult or impossible to maintain a job, or continue with recreational activities like sports or exercise. Friendships and social events drastically reduce in number, and completing errands or making appointments becomes very challenging. Their imaginations run wild, leading to unsolicited or groundless accusations brought about by profound fear and anxiety. These individuals are losing (or have lost) the ability to tell what is real or not.[5]

Schizophrenia: A Case History

We will now walk you through an in-depth case history of a male patient with schizophrenia. This individual was taking multiple medications, yet managed to successfully turn his life around and become drug-free.

Patient Profile

A male patient in his mid-fifties came to me, presenting with a long history of mental illness. The diagnosis, based on the patient's health history, was major depression/anxiety. He had been diagnosed as schizophrenic several years ago and had a family history of similar problems, including general anxiety disorder and PTSD.

The male patient suffered with the following symptoms:

- Chronic depression
- Inability to function normally
- Chronic fatigue
- Severe anxiety
- Suicidal thoughts
- Major sleeping problems
- Nightly cold sweats

- Trouble staying awake
- Very irritable
- High acidic body system
- A very poor diet with many deficiencies
- Excess body weight
- Gallbladder removal (1989)

This patient had gone from being a viable working individual to a non-contributor in society. At work, he started becoming very irritable and falling asleep, ultimately leaving his job. At the point in time that I first saw him, the patient had been off work for 16 months.

The patient's diet was much worse than his spouse had realized. He had been eating sugary candy all day long and spent his days lying on the couch; he also had a frequent craving for ice cream. (Note that sugar always adds to a depressive state, in addition to being very hard on the nervous system and glands. Like other chemical additive drugs or substances, sugar registers as an addictive substance in the pleasure centers of our brain. In other words, the more sugar you eat, the more you will want.)[6]

The patient had great difficulty with focus and attentiveness. During our first two consults, he could not look at me or make eye contact. He looked down and away even when speaking to him directly. Like many similar cases, the patient also experienced chronic fatigue, expressing a desire to play baseball (his recreational sport of choice), but lacking the energy or focus capacity to do so. The patient had also been dealing with 5 years of chronic sleep problems and nightmares. As well, since last year he had been waking up with night sweats, adding to his sleep problems.

Medications
Although it was evident that the patient was continuing to systematically spiral downward over a five-year period, he continued taking the following medications:
- Co-Quetiapine, 100 mg - 2 tablets at bedtime. Co-Quetiapine belongs to the class of medications known as antipsychotics, and is used to treat symptoms of schizophrenia, manic episodes associated with bipolar disorder, and depressive episodes associated with bipolar disorder.

- Teva-Lorazepam, 1 mg - 2 tablets nightly at bedtime and whenever needed. This is an anti-depressant taken for symptoms of excessive anxiety
- APO/Citalopram, 20 mg - 1 every morning. This is an anti-depressant taken to treat symptoms of major depression and anxiety disorders.
- APO/methylphenidate SR, 20 mg - 1 every morning. This medication is **recommended** to treat attention-deficit hyperactivity disorder (ADHD).
- Abilify, 2 mg - 1 every morning. A common medication licensed for the treatment of bipolar disorder, schizophrenia, autism, and major depression (when taken with antidepressants).
- APO/Atorvastatin, 20 mg - 1 at bedtime.
- Ezetrol Ezetimibe, 10 mg - 1 tablet at bedtime. Ezetimibe belongs to the group of medications known as cholesterol absorption inhibitors. It lowers cholesterol levels by decreasing the body's ability to absorb fat.
- Risperidone, 1 mg - 1 in the evening. Risperidone is an antipsychotic medication used to treat schizophrenia and symptoms of bipolar disorder and autistic children. It is an atypical antipsychotic agent for two reasons: first, it is chemically *unrelated* to the older antipsychotic drugs; second, it is *unlike* older antipsychotic drugs.

Problem with Patient's Medications

These classes of medication can act as a type of poison to the brain, interfering with the corpus collasum in our brain, neurotransmitters and brain chemistry. The good news is when the body and brain are supported properly, in addition to the reduction and elimination of medications, over time the brain will develop new neurotransmitters and brain mass. This becomes evident in this patient's changed behavior and symptoms. Depending on the severity and duration of the symptoms and drugs taken, sufficient time for a full recovery must be given. Patience can be greatly rewarded, as seen with this case history; however, protocols must be followed in all recommended areas to achieve optimum results.[7]

Initial Protocol

The following is the recommended treatment plan I prescribed for this male patient, to try and remove the harmful elements in his lifestyle and begin the reversal process.

- Balanced patient's diet. Stopped all sugar except for naturally sweet fruit. Patient's weight reduction was 6 pounds in the first week.
- Vegetable juice daily, standard formula. 1 pint a day (500 ml) or more. (The recipe for this formula, of my own devise, is given below in the dietary food plan).
- Supplements recommended to correct patient's many deficiencies, with special attention to those of brain, thyroid and adrenal support.
- Corrected constipation issues.
- Herbal additions/substitutions for medications taken for anxiety disorders.
- Glandular support, especially the thyroid, adrenal glands, pancreas and pituitary gland.
- Liver cleanse, to improve elimination of drugs, chemicals and fatty substances, especially due to gallbladder removal.
- No coffee while healing. No alcohol, soda or stimulants. No junk food or processed food. Only whole, pure and natural foods/liquids.
- Herbal teas recommended as a beverage or for their medicinal benefit. No limit.
- Supplements were administered to raise/balance dopamine and serotonin levels, as well as hemoglobin levels, in addition to raising the integrity of all body systems and function where needs appeared to be most noted.
- Salt bath, 1 to 2 cups of salt per bath in the evening as a sleep aid.
- An evening walk outside (not in a mall or similarly loud or stimulating environment).
- Daily activity or mind stimulation with a focus/concentration quality required.

Dietary/Supplement Protocol: First Four Months
Supplements were introduced when applicable and added to a juice formula. Unless specified, all supplements were taken with a meal or meal equivalent.

Food could be eaten in addition to drinking fresh juice if desired, with certain restrictions. No processed food/lunch meat, no starches such as bread, potatoes (though sweet potato was allowed), or pasta. Emphasis was placed on raw food, low amounts of animal protein and lots of root and leafy vegetables. It may seem a bit strict, but weight loss was desired by the patient and this diet protocol also increased detoxification of the body and liver.

Snacks included fresh fruit, vegetables, sunflower seeds, pumpkin seeds, walnuts and almonds. Other liquids were restricted to lemon/honey in water, chlorophyll in water/juice, in addition to teas. No coffee, soda or alcohol was allowed, as noted.

The following are the various supplement protocols prescribed to the patient, to be taken over the course of each day at mealtimes.

Breakfast Supplement Protocol
- SAMe on an empty stomach – 200 mg
- Passiflora combo tincture – 10-15 drops, 30 minutes before meals
- Vegetable juice – Made from 2 cups carrots, 1 medium to large beet, 5 leaves of dandelion and sprigs of parsley (1 apple, optional). A protein supplement powder was also added to the juice, along with a tablespoon of hemp hearts.
- Fiber – 1-2 tablespoons ground flax seeds in water just before each meal
- Lecithin granules – 1 tablespoon
- Desiccated glandular extracts – Combination product (1 capsule) plus a pituitary tincture support (10 drops)
- Wild organic salmon oil – 2-3 capsules, 1300 mg per capsule
- Magnesium citrate – 300 mg
- Niacinamide – 1000 mg
- Probiotic – double strength product, 30 minutes after meal
- Kelp – 500 ml (though I now recommend liquid iodine drops 3 times a day, taken on the tongue)

- Coconut oil – 1000 mg
- Vitamin D3 – 2000 IU

Lunch Supplement Protocol

- SAMe on an empty stomach – 200 mg
- 5-HTP – 200 mg on an empty stomach, before meal
- Passiflora combo tincture – 10-15 drops, 30 minutes before a meal
- DHEA – 50 mg
- Vitamin B12 – 1200 mcg under tongue
- Vegetable juice – Made from 2 cups carrots, 1 medium to large beet, 5 leaves of dandelion and sprigs of parsley (1 apple, optional). A protein supplement powder was also added to the juice, along with a tablespoon of hemp hearts.
- Niacinamide – 1000 mg
- Fiber – 1-2 tablespoons ground flax seeds in water just before each meal
- Lecithin granules – 1 tablespoon
- Coconut oil – 1000 mg
- Wild organic salmon oil – 2-3 capsules, 1300 mg
- Kelp – 500 ml

Dinner Supplement Protocol

- 5-HTP – 200 mg on an empty stomach before meals
- Passiflora combo tincture – 10-15 drops, 30 minutes before meals
- Vegetable juice – Made from 2 cups carrots, 1 medium to large beet, 5 leaves of dandelion and sprigs of parsley (1 apple, optional). A protein supplement powder was also added to the juice, along with a tablespoon of hemp hearts.
- Desiccated glandular extracts – Combination product (1 capsule) plus a pituitary tincture remedy (10 drops)
- Niacinamide – 1000 mg
- Magnesium citrate – 300 mg
- Fiber – 1-2 tablespoons ground flax seeds in water just before each meal. Add appropriate supplementation.
- Lecithin granules – 1 tablespoon
- Coconut oil – 1000 mg
- Vitamin D3 – 2000 IU

- Wild organic salmon oil – 2-3 capsules, 1300 mg
- Probiotic – Double strength product, 30 minutes after meal
- Kelp – 500 ml (I now recommend liquid iodine drops, 3 times a day taken on the tongue)

Consumed Any Time

- Juice: 8-12 carrots, 1 medium to large beet, small amount of dandelion and parsley, and 1 apple
- Healthy chocolate (a small amount at one time)
- Liquid chlorophyll, 1 to 2 teaspoons in water at least two times per day

As Needed

- Passiflora combination tincture

At Bedtime

- Valerian tincture – 30 drops
- Flax seed oil – 1 tablespoon
- Salt bath

NOTE: There were more supplements required for this patient, which were given later on to further balance his condition. Initially, this person needed to clear out the toxins in his system from dietary chemicals, drugs and bad fats.

Furthermore, there was the overall challenge to consider. With many patients, even when more supplementation is needed, the patient is reluctant to do so—either due to finances or not wanting to take so many new items at once. In an ideal scenario, I would have added a spectrum of Vitamin Bs, including extra B6, and perhaps something more for tissue cleansing. To help remedy the lack of certain nutrients, the patient also consumed a quality supplement blend with added protein in liquid. Sometimes, things need to be delayed in order to give the patient what will serve best at the time.

Next Four Months: Medication Reduction

- Co-Quetiapine and Teva-Lorazepam (night doses) – Patient gradually stopped taking the night medication in April/May
- Co-Quetiapine, 100 mg – Stopped May, approximant; replaced with herbal tinctures

- Teva-Lorazepam, 1 mg – Stopped May, approximant; replaced with herbal tinctures
- APO – By September, patient reduced *Citalopram* and methylphenidate to 1 every other day (down from 1 per day). His change in mood was noticeable since gradually stopping use of these two drugs. He was having trouble sleeping and complained of "not feeling good". Continued with the program.
- APO/methylphenidate SR, 20 mg – Reduced to every other day from 1 every morning
- Abilify, 2 mg – Patient has never taken this drug, though he was prescribed to take 1 in the morning.

Changes to Patient's Supplement Protocol After Four Months
- Thyroid desiccated extract – 1 capsule 3 times a day with meals
- HTHY (pituitary extract remedy) – reduced to twice a day
- Vegetable juice – reduced to once per day
- B vitamins were included in a combination product, as were several other vitamin/minerals

All other supplement dosages remained the same.

Changes to Patient's Supplement Protocol After Eight Months
Patient still had some lingering unwanted thoughts. The following was added to support dopamine levels and process in the brain.
- L-Tyrosine – 500 mg 3 times per day with food, to be continued for several months before reducing.
  - o Maintenance suggestion: 1 capsule twice a day, which may be reduced to once per day after significant improvement has been maintained for 1 year.
- L-Phenylalanine – 500 mg twice per day with food, to be reduced once enough improvement is noted.

NOTE: Shortly after this time frame, I always start patients of this nature (or those with low thyroid or fatigue) on this quantity of L-Tyrosine.

Patient's Progress After One Year
Within the first year, the patient was off all of his medications. Patient excelled very quickly, applying all that was asked of him, which is remark-

able in and of itself. He lost 30 pounds within the first 5 weeks and has continued losing weight.

Because he was still not working, he did most of the cooking, meaning he always made his own vegetable juice. The patient demonstrated complete compliance with the protocol, which is impressive given the number of lifestyle changes demanded of him. Normally there is more help and assistance required from family members, such as making juice and so on.

He eventually started playing baseball two nights a week and resumed bike riding. His energy has greatly increased as has his metabolism. His zest for life is coming back, as is his integration back into a normal way of living.

The patient felt great overall, but was still dealing with some unwanted thoughts. As stated, patience is required in this process given the time it takes to rebuild new tissue, and remove all chemical toxicity and debris from the brain tissue as well as other areas in the body. The liver typically does not store toxins— it is able to break them down and flush them out— however, toxins can be stored in our fat cells for years, scattered throughout the whole body, including the brain. These toxins in the brain frequently become neurotoxins.

During the month of August, about five months into the protocol, the patient's wife suggested that perhaps her husband could stay on a low dosage of one medication to see if the remaining unwanted thoughts would completely leave. My recommendation was a strong "no"; while I do not force my will on a patient, I will put emphasis on the reasoning behind my recommendations.

My opinion in this case was formed on the basis that the patient and spouse had already experienced the sliding scale of his medication protocol, taken from his previous health history. Add to that the great strides made in all aspects of his health in addition to positive lifestyle changes, and there was nothing to suggest reintroduction of this medication would lead to long-term benefits.

Fortunately, he did not reintroduce the medications once he had weaned off. He, like others of similar circumstance, needed to allow the body sufficient time to fully restore itself.

Current Status (2018)
The patient has stayed with his healthy diet and lifestyle, receiving continued support from his family, and has remained drug-free. This case history

is a wonderful example of what may be possible with patience and trust on the part of the patient and family. Diet and supplementation played a huge role in rebalancing the patient in many different areas of his body, but compliance is also key to making the necessary changes and incorporating a new dietary regime. The patient has continued a daily supportive supplement regime.

It takes great courage on the part of everyone involved when making a transition from a daily routine that has gone beyond the patient and family's control, to one of fighting back to retrieve the person that once was—only healthier. But the benefits of doing so are absolutely worth it.

I do not believe there is any condition that cannot be improved by supporting and enhancing the health of the whole body. As we've said all along, it is all about balance. If you do not feel a sense of balance in your life, it is always to your benefit to seek it out.

CHAPTER 6

Stress and Depression

STRESS CAN BE good for us—acute stress, for example, is meant to help keep us alert and ready for danger—but we don't all respond to stress in the same way. Some experience the symptoms of stress in short, intense bursts; for others, stress persists over extended periods of time. This latter case is defined as **chronic stress**, and it can be a component in developing a major depressive disorder. Whether stress is acute or chronic, certain individuals are more vulnerable to these responses and are therefore more likely to develop major depression.

The heart of the issue lies in the difference between these two types of stress. Both categories of stress response cause overactivity of the adrenal glands by engaging the body's "fight or flight" response; however, chronic stress raises cortisol levels, dampening responses to acute stress. Several other organs and systems are also affected by high cortisol levels, especially the thyroid and adrenal glands, and increased insulin release, weight gain and inflammation can also result.

There are other areas of the body and its systems affected by chronic stress and recurrent depression episodes; most notably, our digestive system, due to the effect stress has on our diet and eating patterns. Those who neglect the need to eat well or supplement their diet with appropriate nutrients to enhance their coping skills can see their diets fall short during periods of stress, leading to nutritional deficiencies that further impact their body's ability to bear up under the increased physical demands of high stress situations.

Bruce McEwen is a brain researcher who heads a neuroendocrinology lab at New York's Rockefeller University. He has spent approximately 50 years studying the way in which hormones and the immune system interrelate during acute and chronic stress in people and animals. According to Dr.

McEwen, "Stress, or being stressed out, leads to behaviors and patterns that in turn can lead to a chronic stress burden and increase the risk of major depression."[1]

Stress Burden

The added burden caused by stress, as well as external circumstances connected to it, together work to overburden the body causing changes in mood and creating physical symptoms.

The following are just a few examples that show the consequences of stress over time:

1. Our brain is greatly impacted by chronic stress, which can result in depression and disrupted sleep patterns, headaches and impaired memory.

2. A continuance of chronic stress levels beyond a person's control results in suppressed functioning in almost all aspects of the immune system.

3. Our reproductive organs and sex hormones are influenced by chronic stress. The risk of miscarriage and increased infertility are associated with chronic stress. Elevated cortisol levels deplete the reserves of the hormone DHEA, involved in the production of sex hormones. As a result, our sex hormones reduce and the libido also begins to decline.

4. Chronic stress has a pronounced effect on our circulatory system, which includes the heart, arteries and veins. Many of us become aware of our hearts racing during acute stress events, but during chronic stress, the circulatory system is still being affected by elevated blood pressure and blood flow to the muscles, putting one at risk of cardiovascular disease or stroke. This prolonged form of stress impedes the oxygenation process that is necessary to keep all the other organs, and the body as a whole, functioning normally.

5. A byproduct of acute and chronic stress, oxidative stress is induced by elevated levels of cortisol. Cortisol is being hailed as the "age-accelerating hormone"; it alters cells at a molecular level by

increasing internal generations of free radicals. Oxidative stress is a key factor in the following conditions: aging, Alzheimer's disease, arthritis, cancer, cardiovascular disease, depressed immune function, endocrine dysfunction, insulin resistance and diabetes, macular degeneration, neurological dysfunction/Parkinson's disease and obesity.

How Do Chronic Stress and Depression Change the Brain?

Using the observational tool of neuroimaging, both depression and chronic stress have been shown to cause structural change in the brain. We touched on how cortisol affects our reproductive system and hormones, but the brain is affected as well: stress and depression cause brain shrinkage in the area that controls our memory (prefrontal cortex). Stress, in and of itself, kills brain cells while cortisol erodes away proper brain functioning.[2]

There are several areas of the brain affected by chronic stress and depression other than the medial prefrontal cortex.[3] Neural systems designed to adjust and modify characteristics of normal emotional behavior have been linked to mood syndromes by evidencing disordered processes (pathophysiology) in the brain. Evidence was compiled from neuropathological, neuroimaging and lesion analysis studies. (For more on the specific brain pathways and precise nutrient requirements involving behavior and emotions, can be found in Chapter 11.)

When discussing the effects of stress on the brain, it helps to have a basic understanding of the many interlinked parts of the brain, and what functions they serve in our cognitive processes.

Medial prefrontal cortex (MPFC). This system is involved with cognitive behavior, personality, expression, controlled social behavior, and even a person's will to live. Dysfunction in the (MPFC) can explain the disruption in autonomic regulation and neuroendocrine responses that are implicated with mood disorders.[4]

Medial and caudolateral orbital cortex. Similar to the MPFC, this area of the brain regulates and coordinates emotional expression. Alterations in grey matter volume and the functioning of the nervous system (neurophysiological) activity are found in cases with recurrent depressive episodes.[5]

Amygdala. An almond-shaped set of neurons which form part of the limbic system, the amygdala is a main player in the processing and experiencing of emotions. This region, like several others, is affected by recurring mood disorder events, leading to shrinkage of tissue and functionality problems.[6]

Hippocampus. An important organ of the limbic system and memory centers, this area regulates emotions and shows volume alterations and function irregularities in repeated depressive incidents.[7]

Limbic and striato-pallido-thalamic structures. This area coordinates emotional expression, memory and arousal (or stimulation) in addition to thinking and movement, and is closely related to the medial prefrontal cortex system. Structural damage in this area is associated with the neurocircuits that underlie depression, evidenced by lesion analysis studies and other brain alterations.[8,9]

Medications Alter Brain Function

In addition to the damaging effects of chronic stress and recurrent episodes of depression, medications used to treat mood disorders and other conditions change our brain structure as well. Of these, antidepressants, psychotics and sleep aids have shown to be the most damaging, causing dementia leading to Alzheimer's disease. Neither are prescription medications exempt from causing brain dysfunction. A few medications have even been spotlighted as causing an increased risk—as high as 54 percent higher—for the development of dementia.

Why are these drugs such a problem? Because these medications store themselves in our body fat, as we age, the processing and detoxifying of drugs slows down due to the health of our liver and kidneys. These drugs continue to accumulate, resulting in an increased occurrence of side effects until one stops taking them for a protracted period of time.

Concerningly, many of the worst offenders are being taken on a regular basis. Now, add to this scenario the lack of nutrition being received by the brain, and you have a recipe for health disasters.

Common Problem Drugs for Brain Health

Drugs commonly prescribed for the treatment of anxiety and sleep problems, as well as antihistamines, have the unfortunate side effect of blocking neurotransmitter activity. Again, neurotransmitters are the chemical messengers of our central nervous system; when they aren't functioning properly, our body can't direct its activities the way it should. In particular, **acetylcholine** is necessary for the processes of learning and memory, and is involved in blood vessel contraction, digestion, circulation/cardiovascular and autonomic nerve stimulation.

For this reason, antidepressants, antihistamines, sleeping pills and incontinence medications have the largest negative brain deficit effect. At the top of the categories listed, benzodiazepines (taken for anxiety, depression and sleep) and anticholinergics (group for allergies and colds) are the worst, increasing your risk of dementia significantly, closely followed by blood pressure and incontinence medications and statins.[10,11,12,13]

Antidepressants and Sleep Aids

Antidepressants, sleep medications and other psychotic drugs are a major cause for concern whenever I see them on a patient's health history. In addition to the risk they carry of stimulating brain dysfunction, they also have a proclivity for having mind altering and personality/character changing symptoms, which continue to escalate the longer an individual remains on this form of medical treatment.

The following is a list of medications to avoid:

Tricyclic Antidepressants

- Amitriptyline
- Amoxapine
- Desipramine (Norpramin)
- Doxepin
- Imipramine (Tofranil)
- Nortriptyline (Pamelor)
- Protriptyline (Vivactil)
- Trimipramine (Surmontil)

For more information on medications that interfere with brain function and how to reverse the ills of dementia and Alzheimer's disease, please see *Reverse Alzheimer's Disease Naturally.*

In the next chapter, we will be covering postpartum depression and insomnia. Since problems with sleep are a constant complaint in patients with mood disorders, having a protocol in place which provides safe alternatives to sleep medication is beneficial; for this reason, we've outlined one such program in the next chapter. This is especially helpful for those suffering with anxiety and certain other forms of depression.

CHAPTER 7

Postpartum Depression and Insomnia

CERTAIN PHYSIOLOGICAL CHANGES take place in a women's body after going through childbirth: specifically, there is a drastic drop in the hormones estrogen and progesterone, which can contribute to a condition called **postpartum depression**. Another main contributor is the health and hormone levels of the thyroid gland, as thyroid hormones also decline sharply after giving birth, lowering copping skills and energy levels. Depression and emotional mood swings present, along with feeling sluggish and even unfulfilled in one's role as a mother.[1]

While all women are susceptible to postpartum depression, when looking at the statistical analysis, we see some gaps. (For various reasons, many cases of postpartum depression go unreported; therefore, these stats only include self-reported cases. As well, these results do not include miscarriages, stillbirths or fetal losses; nor do they take in already existing anxiety or other mood disorders like postpartum psychosis.) In the United States, approximately 4 million births occur each year; of these, 10–20 percent of mothers will experience postpartum depression. Having said that, reports show that 70–80 percent of women do experience some *form* of postpartum-related conditions, at the very least the 'baby blues.' Also indicated is that 50 percent of women experience postpartum symptoms *during* their pregnancy.[2,3]

Including those suffering from stillbirth and miscarriages in addition to cases of postpartum depression, it is estimated that 900,000 women experience postpartum depression annually in the United States. Of these statistics, 1–2 women out of every 1,000 cases will develop a severe form called **postpartum psychosis**, 10 percent of which result in infanticide or

51

suicide. Men also deal with symptoms of depression during this same time frame, at a rate of approximately 10 percent.[4,5,6,7]

Signs and symptoms of postpartum depression include:

- Feeling overwhelmed and hopeless
- Being sad and crying much more than normal for no apparent reason
- Bouts of anger or rage
- Experiencing irritable moods or restlessness
- Constant worrying
- Unreasonable expectations of self or perceived notion of self
- Exhaustion, difficulties with sleep such as oversleeping or not being able to fall asleep
- Brain fog, trouble concentrating, memory problems and difficulty making decisions
- Apathetic, feeling uninterested in activities or circumstances that were once routine or enjoyable
- Appetite is irregular; either eating too much or too little
- Avoidance of loved ones and friends
- Self-doubt in the ability to properly care for one's infant
- Problems bonding with one's child
- Harmful thoughts towards the baby or the mother herself
- Abnormal pain or digestion problems

If left untreated, postpartum symptoms can escalate into a permanent mood disorder. Such instances are very unfortunate, as both the infant and mother suffer greatly, as do other family members. Postpartum can reoccur with every pregnancy, creating more demand for a solution that prevents as well as treats.

Only through whole, natural means can a safe protocol be utilized—one that will not cause more harm or structural brain change. Without treatment, postpartum symptoms will continue to disrupt the mother's health, which in turn affects her care of her baby and their bonding process. The mother could go on to suffer for months or years after the birth, while the baby may develop eating or sleeping problems and behavioral issues as they grow up.

Note that individuals suffering with postpartum depression may be very good at concealing their true feelings and struggles. It is important for spouses, families and close intimate friends to probe a little to ensure all is as it seems. Understandably, *only* certain persons will be allowed into a mother's confidence, and for fear of looking inadequate or being seen as a failure, a spouse may be the last to know. If the telltale signs are there, then measures should be taken and insisted upon to protect all those involved.

Comparing 'Baby Blues' to Postpartum Depression

A high percentage of mothers experience what is commonly called 'baby blues.' As many as 80 percent of new mothers will experience symptoms of increased anxiety regarding their child's care, and issues with fatigue and lower energy, during the first 1–2 weeks after giving birth. This is not surprising given the accelerated hormone usage that takes place during this time period, but these symptoms usually fade on their own.

The symptoms of postpartum depression can be varied and differ between women; therefore, consulting with a health professional would be the best choice for diagnosing this condition.[8,9,10,11]

Treatment Options for Postpartum Depression

Medications for Postpartum Depression

The medications we've discussed so far—with all their attendant problems—are the same ones prescribed to mothers suffering from postpartum depression. These are medications used to alter neurotransmitters in the brain, alongside selective serotonin reuptake inhibitors (SSRIs).[12]

For the many reasons already expressed, the better choice for a treatment protocol would involve treating the chemical imbalances through natural whole sources that support low functioning systems and tissues. These include supplements, diet adjustments and, if needed, natural medicine sources that do not pose a threat to the body and which are non-addicting.

Effective Therapy Treatments

Counseling is a form of talk therapy employed by a variety of professionals such as therapists, psychologists, psychiatrists, counselors and social workers. This type of therapy has shown to be very helpful in the treatment of postpartum depression and other mood disorders. The two forms of counseling that have shown the most promise are cognitive behavioral therapy (CBT) and interpersonal therapy (IPT).

Cognitive behavior therapy (CBT) is a structured therapy dealing with patient's current dysfunctional thoughts (unwanted or negative thoughts) and behavioral problems. This therapy program draws on a wide range of cognitive and behavioral techniques, with the aim being to help people understand their thoughts and reactions to certain situations to effect ongoing improvement in their daily functioning and moods.

The premise of CBT is the evaluation of thoughts and perceptions of that influence a patient's behavior. For example, when a person is feeling overwhelmed and distressed, it can distort their sense of what is real or actually happening. In this instance, cognitive behavioral therapy will help distinguish between what is real while utilizing techniques that provide a solution to a current problem, as opposed to more analytical techniques such as delving into childhood problems, which is customary of traditional psychoanalysis methods.

Cognitive behavioral therapy benefits people of all ages, in addition to helping with many conditions such as the ones discussed in this book and more. CBT has also shown to be successful when delivered online or through in-person therapy sessions.[13,14]

Interpersonal psychotherapy (IPT) centers on current issues and relationships instead of childhood problems. The format of IPT focuses on the patient understanding their responses to psychological symptoms that are occurring in their daily life. In other words, it helps patients to keep a handle on their reactions while working through their personal relationship difficulties.

The therapist plays a very active role, offering many options for changing thought and behavioral patterns. Part of the therapist's function is to offer hope and support while *not* remaining neutral in their role. They help identify any current situation or conflict that may be the source of the distress. They also assist with improving people's communication, interpersonal functioning and social interactions.

This form of psychological therapy is time structured, with typical durations of 12–16 weeks. Interpersonal psychotherapy is performed on a one-to-one basis and in group gatherings.[15]

Exercise

The usual goal when starting an exercise program is weight loss, improved condition, or cardiovascular health. But exercise is also an effective method for improving mental health: studies show how regular exercise greatly impacts depression, stress levels, anxiety and more. Age and fitness level is of no consequence when exercising for stress relief; a person will always feel better after exercising. Once people commit to an exercise program, they notice how much healthier they feel; they sleep better and have more energy.

Studies show exercise lowers depression (mild to moderate), often working as well as antidepressant medications. By keeping up with a regular routine, exercise can also help prevent a depressed person from relapsing.

There are several reasons for why exercise improves stress and depressive moods. A few include the changes that occur in the brain, such as neuron growth, lowered inflammation, the release of endorphins and other specific brain areas involved in good moods, and the calming of nerves.

Exercise also redirects our attention away from negative thoughts, instead focusing on the task at hand. Even breathing during exercise has a positive effect on stress levels and depression. Physically there will be more clarity of thought, improved memory and mental processing, and better physical and emotional well-being.[16,17]

Insomnia

Most people taking medication for depression and sleep have persistent difficulty sleeping. For this reason, we have gathered alternative suggestions that not only help with infrequent sleepless nights or jet lag, but which are especially designed for those who struggle in the early days of stopping their medication, or who report even worse sleep problems during this process.

For far too long, people have been taking the easy way out with regards to their nights of insomnia, turning immediately to over-the-counter sleep medication, all without knowing how addictive sleep medication and some antidepressants are—as well as how much structural brain damage occurs. There are many natural, safe and non-addicting products to choose from instead, for any type of sleep problem. Yet even when patients are made aware of the short-comings of their form of medication, they struggle

greatly in their attempt to stop taking the drugs—often ending up unsuc-
cessful without other intervention.

Thankfully, with nutrient support (to help repair brain tissue/function)
and naturally sourced sleep aids, stopping these medications can be accomplished—as can a good night's sleep. When a body is tired enough, it will
fall into anabolic sleep.

Napping

For some who struggle with falling asleep at night or sleeping through the
night, sleeping in very late in the morning or napping in the afternoon
comes much easier. Of course, this will disrupt normal sleep patterns; if
a body/brain isn't tired enough because it has already rested or is over-
stimulated from mental work or substances taken into the body, you will
not sleep in a healthy or restful manner.

Professionally, I find it interesting how much emphasis is placed on
sleeping for so many hours without waking up. Metabolic nature will
vary from person to person, much of which depends on the health and
function of the person. I've noticed that people who are missing many
key nutrients and have a poor diet can still be good sleepers due to the
fact that their body is exhausted. Other times, the opposite is true: with
proper nutritional support, particularly for the thyroid gland, individuals
may find they need much less sleep than before.

Of course, there are a host of factors which affect our sleep schedules and
ability to fall asleep, many of which have nothing to do with our brain
health. So before we engage a nutritional protocol to help support healthy
sleep, we would do well to make sure our environment is conducive to
good sleep.

State of mind. Most people today are juggling too many duties with
too many demands put upon them, so it should come as no surprise
that when the time comes for the body to wind down from the whole
day's experiences, it's wound too tightly to relax, Some people will sleep
almost immediately, as soon as their head hits the pillow; others will have
difficulty shutting off their minds and will instead obsess over the day's
events.

No need for alarm clocks. Biologically, our bodies will wake naturally when we have rested sufficiently, according or our own individual body's clock. Certain processes and hormones come into play to get us ready for a good night's rest; in other words, we were not intended to work when it is dark. Night shift workers struggle greatly to get adequate sleep during the day, so if you're having persistent sleeping issues, make sure you're sleeping when it's time to do so!

Chemicals and food. It isn't just our work or schedules that keep us up; it is also what we eat and drink. Many are mindful enough of caffeine to avoid taking any too close to bedtime, but there are plenty of people that still take in coffee, tea, soda, nicotine or alcohol close to bedtime. Other stimulants like sugar, white flour products, junk food, chocolate, chemicals in food and other recreational drugs also interfere with normal sleep patterns.

REM sleep. REM sleep is a crucial time of repair and restoration. A major problem with sleep and antidepressant medications is that they bypass REM, despite the fact that it is only during REM sleep that our body gathers collagen and other available nutrients to repair and restore connective tissue, among other important functions.

The bottom line is we cannot function properly without sleep; our body will just continue using itself up. Even though we don't actually require our consciousness to be turned off for the body to rebuild, nighttime is when we see the best restoration.[18] For example, our liver only cleans itself from approximately 1–3 am. This is when the body should remain asleep, but many report waking up routinely from 2:30–3:00 am. It is at this time that our body releases toxins and produces new blood.[19]

Natural Sleep Aids

When seeking to find natural, non-addictive sleep aid, the good news is we already have a wonderful sleep remedy in most of our homes—salt and a bathtub. Three to four cups of salt in a warm bath for 20 minutes in the evening relaxes the nervous system and aids sleep to the point that even those taking sleep medication can discontinue it.

If you try salt baths for sleep aid using this amount of salt, I would suggest a quick shower afterwards to rinse off the salt; however, you can also use lower amounts of salt and see how it works for you. In fact, a bath on its own relaxes and helps prepare our bodies for sleep. For those on sleeping pills and looking to stop, yet feel you will have difficulty doing so, try taking a bath in addition to some of the following helpful suggestions.

NOTE: Any of the following recommendations can be mixed together in any amount that seems to work for you. Herbal tinctures work best and quickest when taken by mouth and held for 30 seconds to 1 minute before swallowing. Follow with supplements or anything to be taken under the tongue, such as melatonin and homeopathic pellets.

For example, you could try mixing two or three herbal tinctures together at bedtime, in addition to taking 9 mg of melatonin, a 30c pellet of the homeopathic coffea, and 300 mg of magnesium—all approximately 45 minutes before bed. (This type of suggestion would be for someone with a real sleep problem, or who is trying to stop medications for depression or sleep.) In such cases, a dosage of herbal tincture would also be taken in the morning and at least once more during the day (or as needed), coupled with other supplements. When taking minerals, either at bedtime or during the day, always eat a small amount of protein if not taken with a meal that naturally contains some.

Once you develop a routine, regardless of the amount of supplements taken, the body will remember your pattern and start to get ready for rest and sleep. For this reason, it is recommended that you take your sleep aids at the same time each day.

- Passionflower: 15–30 drops (¼–½ teaspoon) of tincture on the tongue before bed
- Valerian root: 15–30 drops (¼–½ teaspoon) twice a day and/or one dosage before bed
- Skullcap: 10–20 drops twice a day or at bedtime
- Lemon balm: 20 drops twice a day with valerian root
- Lavender oil: Rub on the temples and place a couple of drops on your pillow (use a pillowcase where an oil stain won't be a problem)
- Melatonin: 3–15 mg under the tongue before bed; start with 3–9 mg and if that's not enough, temporarily take more and then reduce as needed

- As chronic insomniacs may be deficient in B vitamins, Vitamin C, Vitamin D, magnesium, potassium and/or zinc, we recommend the following doses to supplement:
  o Magnesium: 500 mg twice a day or 250 mg three times daily
  o Calcium: 1000 mg before bed
  o Melatonin: 3–9 mg before bed
  o B complex: 100 mg or 2 teaspoons of nutritional flaked yeast twice a day
  o Niacin B3: 100 mg at bedtime
  o Vitamin D3: 2000 IU twice a day
  o 5 hydroxy-tryptophan (5-HTP): 200–500 mg twice a day

Fresh Juice for Better Sleep

Carrot juice mixed with spinach or parsley helps balance the nervous system, which can aid sleep, but that's not all you can do with juicing to help you sleep better. Lettuce juice contains a substance called lactucarium, which acts like a sedative. It also contains a property similar to opium (without the stimulant effects) so those with insomnia should eat lettuce as part of their evening meal. It also has an anti-cramping agent called hyoscyamine.

In addition to lettuce, try to include the following proteins in your evening meal: fish, poultry, legumes, nutritional yeast, and peanuts. These foods also contain Niacin B3, which is involved in serotonin synthesis, which promotes healthy sleep.

Homeopathy to Treat Insomnia

Take two 30c pellets of the following under the tongue and let dissolve if you are experiencing the described issues:

- Coffea: Your mind is awake and working, your brain won't turn off
- Nux Vomica: You're feeling irritable, or experiencing problems with sleeping from stopping sleeping pills, antidepressants, alcohol or food
- Arnica: For physical overwork, can't wind down; jetlag
- Ignatia: Mood swings, emotional distress and yawning frequently

We've discussed the potential negative effects of many of the common medications prescribed for the treatment of depression. However, in this next chapter we will discuss the most common form of self-medication for depression and anxiety—consumption (and overconsumption) of alcohol. Alcohol can significantly affect brain and body function, enhancing depression and anxiety, and even causing death, as alcohol is a poison to the bodies of many genetically compromised people.

CHAPTER 8

Alcohol and Depression

MANY WHO STRUGGLE with symptoms of depression will attest that alcohol relieves their feelings of stress and anxiety. And in small doses, taken infrequently, this may be the case…but what happens when it becomes a habitual remedy, one which then develops into a real dependency?

When it comes to alcoholism and depression an important question is, "Which came first?" In many cases, a person's drinking may have started out as a desire for some 'Dutch courage,' which then became a habit whenever social situations arose, or when they were around new people for the first time. In other cases, an individual may have unresolved personal issues, such as childhood trauma, and lack the skills needed to move forward in life without reliance on substance abuse.

However, in addition to all these possibilities exists another issue: that all mood disorders include some susceptibility to alcohol or drug abuse. When the brain, and the body as a whole, have not been nutritionally supported, imbalances occur, contributing to future mental and physical imbalances. It is for this reason that, when beginning the healing process, it is often a specific nutrient that is most needed to ensure a successful start. For instance, in the case of alcoholism, a B vitamin called thiamine becomes depleted; therefore, it must be replaced for a successful reversal of alcoholism to occur.

That said, there is no one standalone item that acts as a cure all, at least not without sufficient amounts of key nutrients to support the proper functioning of our bodies.

Identifying Alcoholism

When a person drinks heavily using alcohol as a coping mechanism, the alcohol they consume will become a depressant and intensify their feelings of anger or sadness.[1] These issues are made all the more common by how accepted the consumption of alcohol is in North American society, which is the source of many serious problems, from people losing their jobs and families to deaths caused by drunk drivers.

A truly problem drinker can find themselves developing **alcohol use disorder (AUD)**, the symptoms of which include:

- Too much time spent drinking alcohol
- Repetitive drinking patterns of drinking excessively for too long a time period
- Alcohol cravings
- Not curbing drinking even when it is causing problems in relationships and other activities like work
- Limiting time of activities in favor of drinking
- Changing activities in favor of being able to drink while the activity is going on, like fishing or watching sports
- Continuing to drink even when your mood shifts more into depression and sadness
- Not wanting to change your drinking habits even though the link between depression and alcohol is irrefutable

It is reported that about one third of people suffering with major depressive disorder have a co-occurring (mental and abuse problem coinciding) drinking problem like AUD.[2]

Alcohol Abuse Intertwines with Depression

It is not uncommon for people to drink alcohol as their way of dealing with their depression. They might be drawn to its sedative effects; there are other people who may not normally drink, but will use alcohol to help them get to sleep.

Alcohol abuse never leads to a good place. It may seem as though your symptoms of depression have been alleviated, but over time your condition will continue to worsen. In the bigger picture, every aspect of a person's life is negatively impacted by alcohol abuse.

Longer periods of depression will always follow ongoing alcohol abuse. When coupled with antidepressants for those already diagnosed with depression, the depressive effects of the alcohol will worsen the depression and make the medication less effective.[3,4]

How Does the Body Process Alcohol?

Alcohol goes through a two-step process in order to eliminate ethanol from the body. Ideally most of ethanol is processed in the liver, broken down by the enzyme ADH. Alcohol dehydrogenase then converts ethanol into a toxic compound called acetaldehyde (CH3CHO).[5]

Once it turns into acetaldehyde, which is also a known carcinogen, creates problems. Dr. Robert Swift is a researcher and physician who has spent a great deal of time investigating alcoholism at Brown University. He states: "Acetaldehyde is nasty stuff," and that "it's like formaldehyde, which is embalming fluid. It destroys proteins. It destroys DNA." It is hypothesized among scientists that acetaldehyde is the cause of hangovers in all people.[6]

Fortunately, in most healthy individuals (enzyme balanced) aldehyde dehydrogenase very quickly breaks down into the less toxic compound acetaldehyde. Acetaldehyde is then broken down into other compounds like acetate (CH3COO-) which is then broken down into carbon dioxide and water.[5]

However, there are those whose genetic make-up inhibits their ability to break down alcohol, leading to a much greater risk for alcohol abuse. In particular, individuals who either lack or have insufficient amounts of the enzyme alcohol dehydrogenase (ADH), which is needed to process ethanol out of alcohol, are at risk. (For example, North American Indians and 1 in 3 Asians have this enzyme problem, which is why it is not uncommon to hear of a person of North American Indian decent dying from cirrhosis of the liver due to excessive alcohol consumption in their 20s.)[7,8]

Reports show that the liver can process one standard drink per hour—provided the individual possesses normal enzyme levels. When too much alcohol is consumed too quickly, it builds up in the blood and body tissues such as the brain until such time as it can be broken down and processed by the liver.[9,10]

Alcohol Abuse Can Also Lead to Depression

It isn't hard to imagine why a depressed person may be more inclined to turn to alcohol. However, it seems that depression symptoms will continue to surface and worsen from alcohol abuse, according to the National Institute on Alcohol Abuse and Alcoholism (NIAAA). As a depressive state increases, so too does alcohol consumption.

To treat depression that stems from alcoholism, as with most mood disorders, a variety of therapies in conjunction with correcting and supporting nutritional imbalances is the best course of action. Treatment methods would involve Cognitive Behavioral Therapy (discussed on page 54) to prevent a relapse by modifying dysfunctional thinking and behavior patterns. An important benefit to this therapy is in how it prepares a person for the eventual outcomes of problems that may arise, in order to curb their otherwise 'normal' reaction of turning to alcohol. These individuals are in need of better coping skills in addition to nutritive support, and according to the National Institute on Drug Abuse (NIDA), CBT is a highly beneficial therapy in these cases.[11]

Wernicke-Korsakoff Syndrome

If left untreated, alcoholism can progress into a serious condition called Wernicke-Korsakoff Syndrome, a dementia disorder.

Wernicke-Korsakoff is a two-part dementia condition, primarily dealing with Vitamin B1 (thiamine) deficiency. When going without adequate amounts of B1 for a protracted period of time, brain damage can occur, and even fatalities. Note that lack of vitamin B1 not only causes permanent brain damage, but is attributed to several neurological and psychological symptoms.

One of the most common causes of Wernicke-Korsakoff syndrome is alcoholism (absorption problems of thiamine and other nutrients is another causative factor). Other related conditions that can lead to Wernicke-Korsakoff syndrome include HIV/AIDS, widespread cancer of the body, IV therapy over a long period of time without sufficient supplement replacement, and long-term dialysis treatment.

Symptoms of Wernicke-Korsakoff can be divided into two groups. **Wernicke encephalopathy symptoms** involve loss of mental function and proper messaging to muscles, causing leg tremors, as well as problems with vision (such as double vision and unusual eye movements) in addition to alcohol withdrawal symptoms.

A person displaying **Korsakoff syndrome symptoms**, on the other hand, often times makes up scenarios that are not real, along with hallucinations and psychoses and demonstrates severe memory retention problems.[12,13]

Treatment of Wernicke-Korsakoff syndrome normally centers on correcting thiamine deficiency. Previous recommendations were for 100 mg of Vitamin B1 to be taken daily, either orally, intravenously or intramuscularly.[14] However, there has been a change in dosages by the international standards of care and the United States, upping to 500 mg for two to three days (taken intravenous/intramuscular), then reassessing according to noted improvement.[15] If all seems to be going well, the individual continues at 250 mg per day for as long as signs of improvement are sustained. Once a patient reaches a level of stability, 50–100 mg of oral thiamine is recommended to protect against any further neuron damage, especially if a patient continues to consume alcohol or has a problem with a B1 deficiency for any other reason.[16,17]

In addition to supplementing with thiamine, the following herbs and nutrients have been shown to be of benefit: bacopa, sage, turmeric, ginkgo biloba, ginseng, beta-carotene, omega-3 fatty acids and 5-HTP.[18]

After a course of treatment with high-dose parenteral thiamine and reversal of the acute effects of Wernicke encephalopathy, if there is no improvement in the Korsakoff amnesic state or other mental status abnormalities for seven days, then a strategy of secondary harm prevention should be pursued.[18]

We will next be covering how to get started—how to provide yourself with the full body support needed for any successful disease reversal. We'll address in detail the specific nutrients your body earmarks for the areas requiring restoration and rebalancing, in addition to complementary alternative medicines to help deal with any withdrawal symptoms and ultimately replace the need for antidepressant medications.

CHAPTER 9

Complementary and Alternative Health Care

THE UPWARD TREND of complementary and alternative medical therapies shows great promise for the future of health care. In a rather detailed description of natural based treatments put forth in the British Journal of General Practice, it states, "Diagnosis, treatment, and/or prevention which complements mainstream medicine by contributing to a common whole, satisfying a demand not met by orthodoxy, or diversifying the conceptual frameworks of medicine".[1,2]

Led by consumer pressure, there has been an unmistakable rise in complementary medicine awareness and medical research,[3] product brands and their usage,[4] a wider range of available alternative therapies,[5] more insurance providers[6] offering support for these treatments, and the integration of complementary and alternative courses into the majority of U.S. medical schools.[7,8] Non-orthodox and non-pharmaceutical treatments have always been more prevalent in countries other than North America, but are now beginning to make great strides here as well.[9,10,11,12]

Initial Protocol

The goal of natural medical therapy for any illness is to first provide a comprehensive profile of highly bioavailable vitamins, minerals, fats, amino acids, enzymes and antioxidants to support optimal health. To become medication-free, all aspects of body health need to be addressed for the best possible support. For those taking antidepressants, there are predominately 3 areas of protocol. (If a person has yet to take medication for their anxiety, they do not have to go through the weaning off period.)

67

1. Supporting all nutritional deficiencies while reducing all
    unhealthy lifestyle choices.

2. Supplementation to boost coping skills, address nutrient
    shortages, raise energy and create better moods.

3. Medication replaced with natural remedies and supplementation.

Nutrition

Generally, it is best to eliminate all stimulants and 'foodless foods,' including processed foods, as well as substances that lower the immune system (like sugar).

The following are a few foundational guidelines:

- Eliminate white products: sugar, flour, pasta, bread, white rice and potatoes and table salt (small amounts of pink salt daily is beneficial)
- Avoid acidic and chemical-laden liquids and substances: liquid smoke, chemical sweeteners, preservatives, soda, coffee and alcohol
- Concentrate on eating lots of fruits and vegetables. Avoid citrus (except for lemons), eat whole grains like oats and quinoa, wild and brown rice. Prefer root vegetables, sweet potatoes, leafy greens, red, orange and yellow vegetables, nuts and seeds, eggs, fish and the legume family.
- Incorporate fresh juice into your diet. Best choices include carrots, beets and greens for their nutritional value and their inflammation-lowering and cleansing qualities.

Supplements

In general, the most important areas to support with supplements are the nervous system, thyroid gland, adrenal glands, hormone production and the brain. Having said that, many important areas of the body will also be boosted simultaneously by this support, due to the fact that key imbalances in the body will be addressed.

For those who have a known inherent weakness, it is vitally important to always maintain sufficient nutrient levels to avoid system weakness and periods of low energy. For instance, individuals with deficiencies of B12 or iron, when not maintained, will have low energy, lower body functions and reduced oxygen levels. All too often, I see patients not continuing with their supplement regime until a symptom makes itself known, particularly in cases of low blood levels involving B12 or iron.

More detailed information will follow in subsequent chapters about recommended supplements, but as a general overview, the following are valuable in the treatment of mood disorders and supporting full body health.

Omega-3 fatty acids. Derived from fish oil or Super EFAs, the suggested dosage will be higher in natural fish oil products to be sure the individual acquires greater amounts of EPA and DHA properties, when compared to Super EFAs. If inflammation and pain are an accompanying problem, increase dosage to 3–4 times per day until benefit is noticed, and then take accordingly.

Choose from:

- Organic fish oil: 3000 mg twice per day with food
- Super EFAs: 2000 mg twice per day with food

B vitamins. Copious amounts are sometimes needed, so do not skimp on your Bs!

Whole food choices for vitamin B include:

- Nutritional flaked yeast: 1 rounded tablespoon twice per day in liquids or with food.
- B complex formulated for stress: 1–2 times per day with food unless more is required. Some patients will combine flaked yeast with a normal B supplement to boost their daily dosage.
- Vitamin B6 or pyridoxal-5 phosphate (P-5-P): B6 is very important. For those who lack sufficient enzymes to convert B6 into its active form, take 100 mg of P5P with food.

Iodine. Take liquid drops, 5 drops on the tongue 3 times per day. The bottle will typically call for 1 drop three times per day, but in my experience this is not enough to affect noticeable results.

L-Tyrosine. Choose a quality product and take one 500 mg capsule 3 times per day at meals (not late in the evening).

Magnesium. Take 300 mg 3 times per day for bouts of anxiety or when taking several antidepressant medications. Take another dosage at bedtime if sleep is a problem; this dose can be combined with calcium. Take with a protein for best absorption.

Zinc picolinate. Take 30 mg once a day with a meal that includes protein.

Selenium. Take 200 mcg selenium together with 400 IU of vitamin E. Purchase a combination product or buy separately and take these together, one of each twice per day with food.

Vitamin D3. 2000–3000 mg twice per day with food.

Evening Primrose oil. One dose of 500 mg twice per day with food.

Liquid chlorophyll. Take 1–2 teaspoons in 8 ounces of water or add to freshly made juice, and consume twice per day. Sipping throughout the day also works well.

Vitamin C. Take 1000–2000 mg twice per day with food.

Supplements for Major Depressive Disorders

For schizophrenia, bipolar or other severe mood imbalances, you may add the following additional supplements, either one item at a time or together with the listed recommendations.

5-HTTP. Suggested dosage: 500 mg 1–3 times per day with food.

Inositol. Suggested dosage: 500–1000 mg, 2–3 times per day with food. This can be purchased in a powder form, which is helpful for larger dosages. Take with food. (Most brands are available in a powder form, of which ¼ teaspoon is equivalent to 730–750 mg. Depending on the severity of the condition, take ¼–½ teaspoon three times a day.)

L-Phenylalanine: Suggested dosage: 1000 mg 3 times per day with food.

SAM-e: Suggested dosage: 400 mg, 2–4 times a day with food.

Herbal Medicine

When purchasing herbal medicine, here is a good rule of thumb: whenever possible, choose quality products with more potency. Professional practitioners use products with greater potency than the normally available store products; these can be purchased online and from professionals who retail products to their patients. Certain select supplement stores also carry the same products that professionals use.

A brief note on general doses:

- For adults (18 years or older):
    o Dried herbs, 0.5 grams (.5ml/1/8 tsp.) taken 3–4 times per day
    o Capsules/tablets: 2–3 grams, taken 2–3 times per day
    o Tea, 4–8 grams (1–2 teaspoons) of dried herb steeped in one cup of water, 1–3 times per day
- For children:
    o A child's weight must be taken into account when adjusting the recommended adult dose. A typical herbal dosage for adults is intended for an adult's weight of 150 lbs. If the weight of the child is 50 lbs., the appropriate amount would be one-third of the adult dose.

How to Take Herbal Tinctures
Initially, you will want to establish a base dosage that works for your needs. As a general guide, take ½–1 teaspoon of tincture three times per day, starting in the morning.

There are many options for how often these doses can be taken. For instance, to assist in weaning off medications, take herbal extracts a few times a day to better integrate them into your system. These remedies are classified as plant nervines, the source of many medications. You may take as needed, more often and at higher dosages, without fear of addiction. This means more can be taken when episodes occur to help minimize symptoms, especially when there are noticeably less drug benefits than expected.

Similarly, doses may be taken during (or in anticipation of) an anxiety attack. The need for this will differ, based on individual experiences; for example, in cases where there is an ongoing awareness of this disorder, a person might start and end their day with 30 drops of quality tincture.

More may be needed at bedtime to help with sleep, or during a full blown anxiety episode—there are always extenuating circumstances that necessitate a more reactive dosing schedule. In the case of anxiety attacks, as soon as you feel yourself building to an attack, take ½–1 teaspoon (30–60 drops) of quality tincture on the tongue and retain it in the mouth for at least 30 seconds to 1 minute. This enables the solution to absorb into the bloodstream far more quickly, producing quicker calming effects.

Dosage also depends on severity of symptoms, not just frequency or unpredictability. If your symptoms seem overwhelming, continue with 15 drops every 15 minutes for eight dosages, or until relief is felt. You may also use more than one tincture at a time for more support, such as coupling passionflower with skullcap, valerian or St. John's wort. Each of these remedies has something extra to offer; for example, skullcap is especially good for the nervous system and valerian is great for pain.

Alternative Complementary Options

Passionflower tincture. Suggested dosage: 4 milliliters (1:8 ratio) or 20–80 drops, taken 3–4 times per day on the tongue for quicker absorption or in liquid.

St. John's wort. Suggested dosage: 10–15 drops of extract 3–6 times a day (or as needed).

Skullcap. Suggested dosage: 15 drops of extract 3–6 times a day (or as needed).

Ginseng. Suggested dosage: 200–400 mg daily for general preventative medicine. When taken in combination with royal jelly, lifts the spirits and is a great energy booster.

Royal jelly. Suggested dosage: 300–6000 mg per day. Royal jelly is a whole natural food without a definitive dosage recommendation. It can be purchased in powder or capsule form.

Drug and Herbal Interactions

In recent history, there has been a lot of hype surrounding certain medications and their interactions with prescription drugs.

As a practitioner who works extensively with plant extracts, I do not see or experience the adverse interactions being shown in the literature today. This is mainly due to the fact that drugs are so overpowering that they block sensory communication in the body. Plants, in their whole, unadulterated state, do not possess overwhelming isolated compounds that can act similarly to a drug. There *are* known interactions, like grapefruit extract and some vitamin and mineral absorption inhibitors, but in the larger picture any of these contraindications pale in comparison to how medications interfere with the protein pathways in the body. Drugs do not follow the holistic pathway in the body, and thereby interfere with all body functions.

Most, if not all drug and herbal interactions are theory-based. The trials and studies are not taking place. It's not that they shouldn't be, but the variables extant amongst the research subjects present a problem. The studies taking place are typically too small, and the symptoms, medications (including dosages) and plant chemistry need to be the same for accuracy—something that is very hard to achieve in a testing environment.

Do your own investigative work and seek out any full studies being performed on anything you decide to incorporate into your health regimen. I always encourage my readers to form their own opinions and broaden their knowledge base to aid in future decision making.[13]

A Complete Approach is Mandatory

All remedies, whether natural or pharmaceutical, will work significantly better when the whole body has been supported, as we've mentioned several times now. For example, it is more than possible for a type 1 diabetic to reduce their medication or reverse the condition completely while also reducing insulin using natural products (see the case study in the appendix of this book for an example of this).

Our body always works best when functioning as it was designed to—drawing from whole, natural sources that are recognized by the cells in our body, without the imbalance of drug side effects from unrecognizable sources. Yet people are forever in hope of medications being able to solve their health problems. Due to the poor functioning of a weakened body that was never properly supported nutritionally and therefore cannot rebuild itself, this is never a likely result. Mainstream medicine simply does not include addressing the biochemical elements that comprise the body as a whole for optimum function and restoration as part of its protocol.

It should come as no surprise that a tired, weak body will have little possibility of healing itself—when there are too many missing essential elements, proper functioning cannot occur.

The next chapter will follow up on everything we've discussed here, highlighting the application and importance of botanicals with beneficial pharmacological properties. These are remedies that can be used to help you ease off your medications, or even replace them entirely with added support.

CHAPTER 10

Botanicals to Naturally Reverse Depression

L IVING A LIFE that's free from stress is a daydream for most of us. Like it or not, our minds and bodies are daily put through trials, for which we must have sufficient energy and coping ability, lest we end up depleted and drained by the end of the day.

Thankfully, nature has provided a solution and support through numerous healing and adaptogenic plants. **Adaptogens** is a term used to describe plants that support the body by assisting it in adapting to stressors. Fortunately, we live in a time where research has taken big steps forward in uncovering the many medicinal and nourishing properties of plants and other natural sources that we can safely consume.

The following suggestions will assist in all conditions of mild to severe mood disorders, in addition to insomnia and many other ailments.

Ashwagandha (Withania somnifera)

Ashwagandha is synonymous with stress reduction. Ayurvedic medicine has utilized ashwagandha for thousands of years, and it has been extensively researched for its benefits in lowering stress and several other health concerns, such as cardiovascular health. The active ingredient, withanolide, mimics the stress-lowering hormones in our own body. Human controlled trials have shown ashwagandha successfully reduces anxiety and stress disorders, as well as insomnia. Furthermore, some studies revealed that ashwagandha can improve depression.[1,2,3,4]

75

Suggested dosage: To reduce stress and anxiety, a daily dosage of 125 mg to 5 grams for 1–3 months has shown to lower cortisol levels by 11–32 percent. Additionally, 500–600 mg of ashwagandha per day for 6–12 weeks is helpful for reducing anxiety and the onset of insomnia in persons with stress and anxiety. For best results, take for at least one month.[5,6]

Holy Basil (Ocimum tenuiflorum)

There are many reasons why holy basil is so successful at helping those dealing with stress and anxiety ease their symptoms. First of all, every part of holy basil acts as an adaptogenic, assisting the body in adapting to different types of stress while supporting mental balance. For example, the property Ocimum sanctum contained in holy basil decreases stress hormone levels (such as corticosterone), while other compounds like eugenol and triterpenoic acids work to balance hormone levels while displaying preventive effects against stress and reducing the levels to which hormones are elevated during a stressful event. Supportive research also suggests that by taking holy basil twice a day following a meal, types of anxiety associated with depression and stress will be reduced.

Suggested dosage: For curative therapy, take 600–1800 mg daily in divided doses.[7,8]

Rhodiola (Rhodiola rosea)

Only recently in the past decade have American and European researchers been investigating rhodiola as a remedy for depression. However, rhodiola has been studied extensively in Scandinavia and Russia for more than 35 years, but little of the research has been translated into English. Rhodiola, like ashwagandha, is considered to be an adaptogenic, as well as highly safe and well tolerated. Other than several animal trials reporting rhodiola to have antidepressant effects, a human study did report significant patient improvement on the antidepressant effects of rhodiola compared to the placebo group. The study group took 340 mg of rhodiola extract daily for a ten week period.

This herb, like the others in this section, has an outstanding record for reducing stress and increasing resistance to physical and biological stressors. Rhodiola is also beneficial in the treatment of insomnia, fatigue, depression, and hypertension; boosts cognitive performance; cultivates calmness; and enhances the brain's neurotransmitters.[9,10]

Suggested dosage: 200–500 mg, twice a day. If you experience too much energy late in the day that promotes wakefulness, lower dosage.

Passionflower (Passiflora)

Passionflower, similar to the herb valerian, enhances the level of gamma-amino-butyric acid (GABA) in the brain, which calms brain activity and promotes relaxation. Passionflower is one of the most researched herbs in the world, with a long history in traditional medicine. Passionflower is becoming a go-to solution for anxiety, but the list of its applications extends into many areas, from anxiety and pain issues to seizures and hysteria, as well as congestive heart failure and cancer.

Currently, passionflower is primarily used for its sedative and anxiety-relieving effects, either as a single herb preparation or in combination with other plant extracts. Passionflower has been measured against such drugs as Diazepam (Valium), Oxazepam, Lorazepam (Ativan), and Mexazolam, and has displayed equal anxiolytic benefits.[11,12,13]

Suggested dosage: 2–3 grams in tablets or capsules 2–3 times per day. As a tincture, take 1–4 ml (20–80 drops) 3–4 times per day, on tongue or in liquid.

Black Cohosh (Actaea racemosa)

Black cohosh significantly reduced anxiety and depression in multiple studies for mild to moderate mood disorders. This herb is known for its sedative and calmative effects on the nervous system. Black cohosh is also commonly used to treat menopausal symptoms and pain relief.

Suggested dosage: 20–80 mg per day. The product should be standardized to contain 1 mg of 27-deoxyactein. A tincture that equals 2–4 ml can be taken 1–3 times per day in liquid.[14]

Skullcap (Scutellaria lateriflora)

Skullcap has traditionally been referred to as one of the finest nervines and antispasmodics to relieve cramps and relax the body. Skullcap is also a superb anxiety remedy, especially when associated with muscular tension and restlessness. Skullcap has a positive influence on the nervous system, providing a calming yet strengthening effect. For certain symptoms of depression, skullcap is beneficial at relieving headaches, sleepiness and poor concentration.

Skullcap is extremely helpful in acute and sudden-onset panic or anxiety attacks, providing relief without producing a lot of drowsiness. A double–blind study was performed to determine the effectiveness of skullcap for reducing anxiety; in the 19 individuals, skullcap showed significant anxiety lowering capabilities, especially at higher doses. The participants' energy levels and cognition performance were also assessed.[15]

Suggested dosage: Taken as a dried herb, 1–2 grams, 3 times per day. Taken as a tincture, 2–4 ml, 3 times per day.

St. John's Wort (Hypericum perforatum)

The history of St. John's wort as a healing plant has always been impressive. Today, it is mainly called upon for treating anxiety and depression (especially during menopause) and relieving winter blues (SAD). In observing its calming effects on the nervous system, St. John's wort in trials was proven to be more effective than placebo treatment and far better tolerated than antidepressants.[16]

German research has also confirmed its antibacterial effects and shown it to be an excellent remedy for neuralgia when applied externally when compressed to the skin. It soothes burns, heals gastritis and stomach ulcers… the list goes on.

Suggested dosage: Tincture, 30 ml 3 times a day or more often during acute anxiety (up to 2–3 consecutive initial dosages, 30 minutes apart). Dried herb standard dose for depression: 300 mg, 3 times per day.

Ginseng Panax

Ginseng is a shining star of herbal medicine. It maintains the body's equilibrium by monitoring our immune response and our hormonal changes due to stress. For anxiety and depression, ginseng's benefits are twofold: it suppresses the incidence of mental and emotional imbalances of a person as well as prevents stress-related physiological diseases.

Recent research has revealed properties in ginseng involved in the balancing of the hypothalamic, pituitary and adrenal axis (HPA) and the supervision of hormones, thereby producing beneficial effects on the brain, heart and many other areas of the body besides the disease pathways caused by stress.[17,18]

Ginseng is traditionally used in Japan, China, Korea and North America as a medicinal herb.[19] Ginseng's pharmacologically active compounds found in its leaves, roots, fruit and stems are well known and established.[20] These pharmacological elements have shown to support many brain compartments including neuronal growth, synapse and neurotransmission, all the while protecting our central nervous system from unforeseen events.[21,22] Ginseng's long list of accolades is extensive, however particularly relevant is its ability to reduce the disproportionate inflammatory response in acute and chronic inflammation, which can result in damage and impaired body function.[23]

Suggested dosage: For treating conditions of depression and anxiety, a minimum dosage of 400 mg of extract daily and 200–400 mg as maintenance is suggested. Other suggestions include a preparation of crude dried root powder, 1–2 g taken daily for up to 3 months. In scores of clinical studies, the dosage of crude root ranged from 0.5 to 3 g per day; the dosage of extracts normally ranged from 100–800 mg.[24,25]

Schisandra (Schizandra chinensis)

Schisandra, like so many herbal recommendations found in this section, imparts a wide range of benefits. Because schisandra is an adaptogen and a hormone balancer, it is very useful in the treatment of anxiety, stress, and fatigue, and works as an antidepressant, immune booster and liver detoxifier.

Schisandra is commonly used in traditional Chinese medicine as a liver and blood purifier and as a preventive for adrenal fatigue. Besides these benefits, schisandra also assists in fighting cardiovascular disease through its high antioxidant concentration (fighting free radicals), which lowers inflammatory immune responses. By lowering inflammation via the immune system, schisandra has been shown to inhibit the development of atherosclerosis while also balancing blood sugar.

Suggested dosage: Taken as a tincture, 20–30 drops per day. Taken as a fruit powder extract, up to 3 grams per day. Taken in capsules/pills, 1–3 grams per day with a meal.[26]

Valerian (Valerianna officinalis)

Dating back to ancient Greece and Rome, valerian root has been used as a medicinal tea. Valerian contains a number of different alkaloids and compounds, of which the most noted would be gamma-aminobutyric acid (GABA), long known as a remedy for depression, anxiety, and insomnia. Valerian has shown to be non-sedative.[27]

GABA is a naturally occurring amino acid that induces relaxation by blocking stress instigating chemicals (neurotransmitters) in the brain. The same chemical that is activated when taking the drugs Xanax and Valium is the one found in valerian root; i.e., GABA. Valerian offers a number of benefits including lowering blood pressure, calming nerves, regulating heart rhythms, and strengthening the heart, and can treat insomnia, ease pain, and even help with impaired breathing. Valerian is also recommended for nervous dyspepsia (stomach and intestinal cramps), among other abdominal pain issues.[28,29,30]

Suggested dosage: Take as tincture, 2–4 ml as needed for anxiety (try 2 ml, 3 times a day).

Lemon Balm (Melissa officinalis)

Lemon balm has a pleasing taste that is suitable for children and adults. It is best known as a mood lifter, and yet current research points to its having antidepressant properties, as was revealed by the British Psychological Society in April 2004. It has shown to be very supportive to the nervous system during stressful episodes.[31]

Suggested dosage: For adult depression, higher dosages are recommended for optimal effectiveness, with the lowest dosage recommendation being 300 mg. Amounts 3–4 times this minimum proved much more beneficial in studies.[32]

L-Theanine

L-Theanine is extracted from green tea and is widely used in the treatment of depressed moods and anxiety throughout many Asian countries. Studies have revealed that L-Theanine increases the levels of several neurotransmitters in the brain with general neuroprotective effects. Examples include dopamine, serotonin and gamma-amino-butyric acid (GABA).

Generalized anxiety responds to a 200 mg dosage of L-Theanine and may work for more severe symptoms, although for more extreme symptoms a dosage of 200 mg taken every 3–4 hours would prove more beneficial.[33]

Herbal medicine, while being effective at managing stress, can't do it all. If your lifestyle is one that constantly places you in stressful situations, you will need to explore the possibility of making small but effective lifestyle changes to better cope with your anxiety. Even a small change in your daily routine to incorporate de-stressing activities and physical exercise can work wonders.[34]

CHAPTER 11

Nutrient Support for Reversing Mood Disorders

WHEN A PERSON finds themselves in a state of persistent fatigue or depression, often their endocrine system and brain are to blame. Both of these conditions require support from specific hormones and particular glands and organs of the endocrine system, support that can be greatly aided or enhanced by supplementing with whole plants or their concentrated extracts *and* specific nutrient support required for function and repair.

Yet with today's less-than-optimal agricultural practices, it is nearly impossible to nutritionally provide what the brain and body require from diet alone. Extra supplementation of certain nutrients has been proven necessary to ensure adequate performance and disease prevention. In this chapter, we will look at a few nutrients required to support the intricate pathways in our brain that monitor our emotions and cognition, a delicate system that easily starts malfunctioning when specific nutritional elements are not provided.

Dopamine

The neurotransmitter **dopamine,** supported by other neurotransmitter precursors, promotes balance in the brain and emotional wellness. There are a few essential nutrients related to cognitive function and dopamine neurotransmission, including: marine omega-3 fatty acids, vitamin D3, folate (5-MTHF), L-Tyrosine, B6, pyridoxal 5 phosphate (P5P), zinc and other supporting nutrients.[1,2,3]

But first, a brief overview as to how dopamine is produced and utilized by the body. Having this understanding will be helpful in following how and why our body needs specific nutrients to carry out its normal business.

The process begins with phenylalanine, a precursor for the amino acid L-tyrosine, and the monoamine neurotransmitters dopamine, epinephrine (adrenaline) and norepinephrine (noradrenaline), among others.

This precursor becomes L-Tyrosine, which is then converted to L-DOPA by tyrosine hydroxylase (TH), a function which requires active folate (5-MTHF). This form of folate easily crosses the blood brain barrier. Adaptation of L-DOPA to dopamine is then intervened by the amino acid decarboxylase (AACD), a process which calls for the active form of B6 (pyridoxal 5 phosphate (P5P).

Dopamine is then released into the space between two neurons (into the synapse), which is how we describe communication between neurons. Through this action, dopamine now binds to dopamine receptors by way of the receiving neurons (postsynaptic).

At the site of the dopamine receptors, the message is translated to support cognitive functions. If dopamine remains in the synapse, it may be re-taken or degraded by two enzymes called monoamine oxidase (MAD) and catechol O-methyltransferase (COMT).

Other nutrients are involved as supports in this process, with polyphenols protecting neuronal/brain function and health, and zinc offering significant support for positive mood and behavior and maintaining healthy cognitive function. Supporting or supplementing these nutrients aids this entire process, which results in raised dopamine levels and improved mood.

Important Nutrients for Brain Health

Vitamin D and Marine Omega 3 Fatty Acids

Vitamin D and omega-3 fatty acids play a significant role in all mood disorders and behavior because they control serotonin synthesis and action. Yet 70 percent of the population has inadequate levels of vitamin D and low levels of omega-3 fatty acids, meaning serotonin synthesis will not be optimal in these individuals. Cell membranes depend on fatty acids for membrane fluidity, a crucial cell function. Marine omega-3 fatty acids influence the action of serotonin by enhancing membrane fluidity, which increases the serotonin receptors' ease of access to postsynaptic neurons (message receivers).

The Nutrition and Metabolism Center, Children's Hospital Oakland Research Institute in Oakland, California reported on the outcome of supplementing vitamin D and omega-3 fatty acids (specifically two marine omega-3 fatty acids, eicosapentaenoic acid (EPA) and docosahexaenoic acid (DHA)). Eicosapentaenoic acid (EPA) in particular increases serotonin release from neurons before the synapse (presynaptic) by reducing prostaglandins (E2 series), and is involved in a wide range of body functions such as modulation of inflammation, dilation, control of blood pressure, constriction of blood vessels and muscles, and more.

Initially, they noted from previous findings that serotonin regulates sensory gating, social behavior and executive functioning. A commonality was shared in the defects of these functions, with that of bipolar disorder, schizophrenia, attention deficit hyperactivity disorder and impulsive behavior. Researchers are still exploring the reasons why supplementing with omega-3 fatty acids and vitamin D improves cognitive function and behavior in these brain disorders, but the importance of their results supports the need to incorporate these supplements into any treatment plan for mood disorders or cognitive illnesses.[4]

Researchers Patrick, R. P. and Ames, B. N., suggest, "We propose a model whereby insufficient levels of vitamin D, EPA, or DHA, in combination with genetic factors and at key periods during development, would lead to dysfunctional serotonin activation and function and may be one underlying mechanism that contributes to neuropsychiatric disorders and depression. This model suggests that optimizing vitamin D and marine omega-3 fatty acid intake may help prevent and modulate the severity of brain dysfunction."[5]

Tryptophan
Brain serotonin is synthesized from tryptophan, which then transfers genetic information to the body's messenger RNA transcriptionally when activated by vitamin D hormone. Low levels of vitamin D therefore affect this function.

Sufficient levels of Vitamin D and eicosapentaenoic acid (EPA) are required for normal tryptophan metabolism. When the body has adequate amounts of these two nutrients, we then see an increase of tryptophan hydroxylase 2 (TPH2), which is required to produce serotonin (5HT);

meanwhile, sufficient levels of (EPA) enable 5HT to be released by means of the presynaptic neuron. Docosahexaenoic acid (DHA) plays an important role in this metabolic pathway as well; for the binding of 5HT to the serotonin receptor (5HTR) to occur in the postsynaptic neuron, sufficient amounts of DHA need to be present.

A lower level of vitamin D inhibits the production of tryptophan hydroxylase 2 (TPH2) which in turn results in a much lower production level of serotonin. When all the steps in this process are properly supported with adequate nutrient levels, normal serotonin neurotransmission can occur, which allows for executive function, sensory gating and prosocial behavior.

A special note on postpartum and postmenopausal cases, both instances when women have lower levels of estrogen which encourage mental illness like bipolar: there are specific estrogen levels associated with lower levels of omega-3 fatty acids and vitamin D that lead to mental disorder vulnerability in women.[6] During these biochemical changes, there is an abrupt drop in estrogen levels (between 100 and 1000) during the first four months of postpartum and below 30 pg/ml for women postmenopausal (with normal levels before menopause ranging from 30–400 pg/ml).[7,8,9]

Folic Acid

In a clinical study performed at the Harvard Medical School, Dr. Fava, director of the depression and research program, found that patients with low folate levels had a much lower response to antidepressants than those with normal levels.[10]

In several studies looking at two commonly prescribed antidepressant medications, L-methylfolate was found to improve the efficacy of serotonin reuptake inhibitors (SSRIs) and serotonin-norepinephrine reuptake inhibitors (SNRIs). The initially lower dosages of 7.5 mg for the first 30 days showed little benefit, but when the dosage was doubled to 15 mg/day for the next 30 days, L-methylfolate showed significantly greater efficacy compared with subjects on continued SSRI therapy.[11,12]

And even though folate can be found in grains, beans, fruit and vegetables, for many people supplementing with folic acid has shown to be the better option, as it is more rapidly absorbed by the body than folate. There can still be problems with absorption even with folic acid due to intestinal diseases or other organ disease involving the liver or kidneys *or* genetic mutation of L-methylfolate. (Other inhibitors include pregnancy, excessive alcohol consumption, eating disorders and certain medications which affect the absorption of folate.)[13]

To ensure better absorption rate, L-methylfolate is the more easily bio-available form of this supplement. For a therapeutic dosage, consider 400 mcg daily (or perform a blood test for exact requirement).

Lithium

The pharmaceutical drug form of lithium, which is marketed under the brand names of Eskalith and Lithobid, comes with a long list of brain and body-damaging side effects. For those on additional or multiple medications, the medication lithium has *serious* interactions with at least 75 other drugs, *moderate* interactions with at least 134, and *mild* interactions with at least 64 different drugs. For this reason, the mere mention of lithium should set off alarm bells, not the least of which due to this drug's frequent association with bipolar disorder.[14,15,16]

However, the trace mineral variety of lithium, which naturally occurs throughout our body, belongs to the same family of minerals as potassium and sodium and is beneficial for cognitive function.[17] Studies have shown that lithium increases cortical thickness (thinner and smaller grey matter mass) in bipolar patients,[18] can be a viable treatment strategy for conditions from mild brain impairment to dementia and Alzheimer's disease, and can help treat acute brain injuries and other chronic neurodegenerative diseases.

Lithium (the natural, or **orotate,** version) should be taken at a very low dose as a daily supplement. A highly beneficial aspect of lithium orotate is that it passes the blood brain barrier much more effectively than other forms, making it especially good for anxiety, depression and emotional balance, and over a long term can enhance bone density and cognitive execution and even increase lifespans. Other related benefits include increasing the activity of stem cells and the number of mitochondria, as well enhancing the transport of folate and B12 into cells, all of which can potentially provide additional brain protection. Furthermore, it increases cellular waste (autophagy) including damaged proteins[19] while also reducing tau induced tangles, common in chronic dementia disorders like Alzheimer's disease.[20,21,22]

Lithium is traditionally harvested from mineral springs and brine pools, in addition to being mined from igneous rock. Lithium orotate is a salt derived from orotic acid, while lithium aspartate is sourced from aspartic acid, an amino acid. Both of these forms are available as over-the-counter purchases; overall, orotate is the better choice, as aspartate is thought to be an excitotoxin, meaning a substance that binds to nerve cell receptors, and which may induce overstimulation, causing headaches, inflammation, and brain edema along with nervous and vascular system problems (especially in sensitive people).[23,24]

Lithium concentrate is found in crustaceans and mollusks, and in low amounts in fish like scallops, oysters, clams, shrimp and lobster. Fortunately, lithium can be generously sourced from the legume family—in particular soybeans, beans, lentils, chickpeas and dried peas. Generally, vegetables have significantly less lithium, with the exception of sea kelp, blue corn and mustard seeds, all of which still only provide trace amounts. Small amounts of lithium can be found in grains like wheat and rice, in pistachios, and in dried fruit and coffee.[25]

However, it is imperative to nutritionally care for your thyroid gland when taking lithium. Even though this form of lithium is far removed from its drug counterpart, remember to take iodine and other essential nutrients outlined in Chapter 12 for optimum gland and body functioning. I suggest starting with a low dosage of lithium orotate, especially when coupled with other beneficial and balancing supplements and other herbal medicine. Avoid high dosages of lithium, as there could be serious health risks.[26,27]

As a dietary supplement, any dosage below 5 milligrams is safe. A typical dosage falls between 0.3–5 milligrams to boost brain protection, on up to 15 mg for stronger symptoms of anxiety and other depressive disorders (which may also come with symptoms of sedation). At this dosage level (15 mg), there are definite anti-anxiety and anti-depression effects.

S-Adenosylmethionine (SAMe)

SAMe is an intrinsic component of our mental and physical well-being, possessing an extensive list of benefits. Biochemically, SAMe is formulated in the body from methionine (amino acid) and is a required element for the production of adenosine triphosphate (ATP). It is found in greatest concentrations in our brain and liver and is vital to our metabolism. It is also essential for production of our body's most important antioxidant glutathione, as well as some secondary antioxidants. Studies have revealed SAMe boosts the levels of dopamine, serotonin and norepinephrine, providing antidepressant support.[28,29]

SAMe is normally available in two forms: a butanedisulfonate form and a tosylate form. Richard P. Brown, M.D. an associate professor of clinical psychiatry at Columbia University College Physicians and Surgeons, has made use of S-adenosylmethionine for years in his studies and has since progressed into other complementary alternative medicine in the treatment depression. He suggests looking for SAMe in the form of butanedisulfonate, as he has found it to be more helpful, especially in the enteric coated form. This form allows the supplement to bypass the stomach's acid and open up in the small intestine, for maximum benefit.

Regarding dosage, there are many studies that recommend varying dosage amounts. Here is one example reported by Dr. Brown using a higher dosage: "Rapid response to SAM-e was shown in a double-blind trial of 30 depressed in patients who received either 1600 mg/day of oral SAM-e or imipramine (averaging 140 mg/day) for six weeks. The SAM-e group was significantly better by day 10. Both groups were comparably improved by week 6."[30,31]

I suggest starting with a lower dosage for one week before increasing to higher levels, especially when partnered with other suggestions in this book, as less may be needed. As a guide, take 400 mg for mild depression, starting with 200 mg taken 30 minutes before a meal such as breakfast and lunch (rather than before dinner in case of any stimulation effects).

Magnesium

Low levels of magnesium can lower serotonin levels in the brain, but we hardly need another reason to supplement magnesium in our bodies. There isn't anyone who wouldn't benefit from more magnesium—it is one of the most crucial elements in the body![32]

There are many studies linking magnesium levels to mental health and stress syndromes. All biological aspects of depression are impacted by the presence (or absence) of magnesium in the nervous system. Like glutamate and calcium, magnesium hangs about in the synapse between two neurons, but magnesium actually guards against glutamate and calcium continually activating N-Methyl-D-aspartic acid (NMDA) receptors, which can otherwise result in damage to neurons and eventually cell death. If magnesium is deficient in the body/diet, there is no neuron protection taking place during this process.[33]

Magnesium also suppresses the ability of the hippocampus to stimulate the stress hormones adrenaline and cortisol by slowing down the release of adrenocorticotropic hormone (ACTH). The ACTH hormone regulates the levels of the hormone cortisol being released from our adrenal glands.[34] We know that chronic stress leads to excess cortisol, which will in due course result in damage to the hippocampus followed by negative responses that then continue to produce ongoing depression, stress and neurotoxicity.

Zinc

Like magnesium, zinc is another influential element without which we cannot remain healthy. As with magnesium, zinc holds a long list of important tasks and is found in the highest concentrations in the brain's hippocampus. Research has shown that those suffering with depression tend to have low serum levels of zinc, with the more severe their depression, the lower their zinc levels. Deficient serum zinc contributes to ADHD, poor memory and learning problems aggression and violent behavior, seizures and worsening symptoms of depression.

Low levels of zinc create more inflammation throughout the body, because the T-cells of our immune system cannot function without zinc. Yet when our bodies are under chronic stress conditions, zinc is quickly secreted via our urine, perspiration and saliva. Although supplementing zinc alone is not the answer to depression, it *can* go a long way in aiding someone's recovery.

Suggested dosage: Take zinc picolinate (a more absorbable form) 30 mg, twice a day with 2 mg of copper with a meal that includes protein. As improvement is felt, reduce to once a day unless falling ill to respiratory illnesses or gut diseases like colitis or Crohn's disease, or other chronic diseases or ongoing health problems. Too much zinc on its own without copper creates a copper deficiency; for this reason 50 mg of zinc taken in one concentration would be too high without a copper complement.[35,36]

Medium Chained Fatty Acids

Medium chained fatty acids (MCTs) contribute to the balance of hormones and our brain's need for a constant energy source to maintain proper function. Medium chained fatty acids MCTAs go straight to the liver for processing, unlike longer chain fatty acids where, depending on the body's need, they will either be turned into ketones or be used as an immediate energy source.

MCTs are particularly helpful when blood glucose is low, which then stimulates the liver to break down stored fat to produce ketones. Ketones are the brain's preferred food source, even over any available glucose. So, by supplementing with MCT oil, you can significantly raise the levels of ketones that can easily cross the blood brain barrier, immediately boosting energy to the brain. Lastly, medium chain fatty acids do not require carnitine for beta-oxidation, unlike long chained fatty acids (which are carnitine dependent).[37,38]

Collectively supporting the body's hormones and brain health warrants MCTs be used as a preventive part of a treatment plan to remedy depressive disorders and all cognition impairment. Medium chain fatty acids are naturally found in greater amounts in coconut oil, clarified butter (ghee), palm oil and cheese. Today, MCTAs are also readily available as a dietary supplement, commonly found in liquid form or capsules.

Suggested dosage: Take as a supplement in oil form, 2 teaspoons twice a day near a meal.

Phosphatidylserine

Phosphatidylserine is an amazing fatty substance called a phospholipid which protects and covers the cells in our brain. It is important for the preservation of our mind and memory sharpness and intelligence.[39] Deteriorating mental health and memory problems are closely related, and phosphatidylserine has been shown to help both mental health and memory problems.[40]

Rather than directly impacting the hormone serotonin, phosphatidylserine works with other brain friendly supplements to enhance their effectiveness. For example, curcumin (discussed below) increases blood flow in the brain and also stimulates the production of serotonin and dopamine. Yet curcumin has problems with its low absorption rate. Phosphatidylserine lends a helping hand in improving curcumin's bioavailability.[41]

Curcumin

Curcumin, a primary bioactive compound in turmeric, protects our brain in many impressive ways. It raises levels of dopamine and serotonin, while also increasing blood flow to the brain; it's also a potent antioxidant and anti-inflammatory, reducing the brain inflammation associated with depressive disorders.[42,43]

A double-blind placebo-controlled study of 56 persons with major depressive disorder (MDD) was published by Adrian Lopresti, PhD, of Murdoch University, Australia, in June 2014. The study took place over an eight-week period during which supplemental curcumin resulted in reducing overall indicators of depression, including reducing symptoms of anxiety. Dr. Lopresti reports, "Curcumin's positive antidepressant and anti-anxiety effects are likely due to its ability to normalize specific physiological pathways. It appears to elevate neurotransmitters such as serotonin, while lowering stress hormones, such as cortisol, and is a potent antioxidant and anti-inflammatory. Curcumin also provides protection to the brain."[44]

Astaxanthin
Astaxanthin (AST) demonstrates its benefit through its well-documented immune and anti-inflammatory stimulating effects. Astaxanthin possesses the ability to cross the blood brain barrier, and helps in reducing oxidative stress—known to impact psychiatric disorders like depression and anxiety.[45]

Found in many aquatic species, astaxanthin is a fat-soluble red carotenoid which has gained notoriety for its enhanced ability to protect the nervous system, brain and eyes. Astaxanthin is also gaining popularity due to its unique characteristic that, when recycling free radical electrons, astaxanthin does not become ineffective, even after eliminating these extra electrons. Astaxanthin is therefore one of the most powerful carotenoids, given the unique way it protects plants, animals and sea life.

Suggested dosage: 4–10 mg, taken twice per day.

CHAPTER 12

Supporting the Thyroid and Adrenal Glands

NO TREATMENT PLAN for a depressive disorder will be successful without sufficient support given to the thyroid and adrenal glands. Both systems play prominent roles in the stress response and all related mood syndromes.

The thyroid gland is *the* crucial component for regulating our body's efficient energy production throughout the day. When a thyroid condition presents, or the thyroid is found to be underperforming, certain nutrient deficiencies are always a prime suspect. Prolonged imbalance can result in a hyper thyroid state or other thyroid anomalies, which can in turn lead to loss of function throughout the body as energy production slows down. (There is also a developing problem in North America related to leaky gut, or intestinal diseases, and the ingestion of gluten, which is causing an auto-immune condition affecting thyroid health called Hashimoto's disease.)

The adrenal glands are small, grape-sized glands that lie on top of the kidneys. You can think of them as our body's "shock absorbers", as these very hard-working glands are responsible for regulating our body's response to stress. The adrenal glands consist of two main sections, described as the outer adrenal cortex and the inner adrenal medulla. The adrenal glands also have a direct line to the brain (the medulla), unlike other glands whose messages are related solely via hormone pathways.

The relationship between the thyroid and the adrenal glands is closely intertwined; so much so that when the adrenals become exhausted or lose functionality, there is a direct negative effect upon the thyroid gland. For this reason—and others relating to our total body perspective on disease reversal—it is imperative we look after this area of our endocrine system and restore these glands as necessary to achieve optimum health and function.

Supporting Thyroid Health

Stress impacts our thyroid and endocrine function in a number of ways, but it is only when the demands placed upon us exceed our ability to cope that we find ourselves on the path to anxiety and depression. When these circumstances become chronic and constant, the body cannot help but start to buckle under the constant bombardment of high levels of cortisol and corticosterone.

In these circumstances, one of the best things you can do (besides making lifestyle changes to minimize incidences of avoidable stress) is to give your body all the nutritional support it needs.

This is made more necessary because the cells in our body cannot differentiate between foods and substances that promote cell *energy* or cell *exhaustion*; our cells don't know what's best for them, so the responsibility falls on us to make great food and quality supplementation choices that will both produce and sustain our vitality. Remember: diet is the best tool we have in overcoming a vast number of emotional and physical illnesses.

But like most things that involve change, it takes practice to develop self-control and build a new routine, whether it's taking a few supplements on a daily basis or making a point to add something new and healthy to your diet. Know that your body and brain *will* work with you to help you stick to new, healthier choices; the longer you apply yourself, the easier it gets!

Diet and Supplement Suggestions for Thyroid Health

Nutrients that are critical for thyroid function and its production of T4 include iodine, tyrosine, chromium, selenium, and zinc. When these items become unavailable (whether through diet or just because they are present in very low supply), thyroid function will be diminished. A few other reasons for why someone may be lacking in these nutrients, other than an inadequate diet source, include: gastrointestinal problems, the use of oral contraceptives, low acidophilus/bifidus organisms, or a diet high in processed foods (as food processing easily destroys these nutrients). By adding quality supplements or herbs to increase our intake of mineral and vitamins, we can help ease these various deficiencies. However, your endocrine tissue and brain also require high quality fat and protein, in addition to specific nutrients to boost certain hormones. The following are some general guidelines for what to do (and not do) to support your thyroid's health.

Avoid Sugar and Caffeine

Whether your thyroid condition is hypo or hyper, it's best to avoid sugar and caffeine products. Often, people with low thyroid condition turn to these stimulants to compensate for their lack of energy…but what they don't realize is the harm being inflicted by high amounts of caffeine and sugar. In general, eat less starchy foods, carbs, sugar, and sugar products (unless they're deemed safe, as for a diabetic) and eat more non-starchy vegetables and greens. For hyperthyroidism, avoid all refined foods, dairy products, wheat, gluten, sugar, caffeine, coffee, alcohol, and other chemical stimulants.

This is particularly pertinent given that we're discussing the treatment and prevention of mood disorders. For all the current buzz about the opioid crisis, we overlook the addictive qualities of the sugar we add to nearly all our food! Sugar is highly addictive and brings about anxiety, depression and mood swings. The opioid receptors located in the brain and the spinal column (seven transmembrane-spanning, G protein-coupled receptors), responsible for assisting our neurotransmitters and hormones (in particular our endorphins) are made to go haywire by the way addictive substances act upon these sites.

A few sugar alternatives include raw honey, maple syrup, stevia, agave, blackstrap molasses, and brown rice syrup. For a low-glycemic choice that isn't artificial, stevia has no effect on blood sugar and is devoid of calories. Raw honey is acceptable when used in moderation.

Prioritize Best Fats and Proteins

The importance of including the right fats in your diet cannot be over-stated, with special emphasis on your intake of omega-3 fatty acids in the form of fish oil and seed oils (such as flax seed). Your glands require high quality protein and fat to work properly. Other good fat sources include nuts and nut butters, avocados, seeds (like flax and sesame), olive oil, ghee, coconut oil and milk products, full fat and aged cheese, yogurt, kefir, and cottage cheese.

Adequate quality protein sources also benefit thyroid and adrenal gland function, as protein transports thyroid hormone to the tissues. Choose drug-free flesh proteins and vegetarian sources such as legumes and nuts, seeds, and butter made from the same.

Probiotics

Another essential dietary component for health maintenance and proper functioning of the thyroid gland is the consumption of probiotics in supplement form, or else in certain foods such as yogurt, kefir, and clabbered milk. Twenty percent of thyroid gland function depends on friendly flora!

A special word on soy, as soy products are often touted as a dairy replacement. Soy has made the list of the eight most significant food allergens, as put out by the Food and Agriculture Organization of the United States. People with thyroid and autoimmune thyroid disorder conditions should consider avoiding soy, especially if you are sensitive or allergic to soy.

Remember: if you are simply sensitive to a food or substance, you may not see a reaction for several hours or even a couple of days, while an allergic reaction is usually immediate.[1,2]

L-Tyrosine

The amino acid tyrosine is classified as a "nonessential amino acid" derived from the amino acid phenylalanine. It is, however, essential for the production of several neurotransmitters (brain chemicals) including dopamine, epinephrine and norepinephrine.

L-Tyrosine is an amino acid earmarked for the thyroid gland which, during times of under-activity, offers more than one benefit. Most often, amino acids are tied into the neurotransmitters of the brain. In the instance of L-Tyrosine, it is a required element for dopamine and a neurotransmitter responsible for any number of functions, including mood and sleep. Increasing the health of the thyroid, then, has a direct effect on one's emotional well-being—a victory, all round.

Because tyrosine is the precursor of the neurotransmitters dopamine (DA) and norepinephrine (NE), which play a part in the brain's response to acute stress, supplementing L-Tyrosine helps improve mood disorders. Researchers are currently looking into tyrosine as a treatment option for depression, and overall, many studies suggest using L-Tyrosine as an antidepressant.[3,4,5] Personally, when treating patients for all manner of depression, as well as ADHD and mental disorders like bipolar and schizophrenia,

L-Tyrosine is a main feature of my treatment plans. Most patients see noticeable improvement in one week's time.

Tyrosine is also a main component in our body for making energy.[6] Chronic depression, exhaustion and poor metabolism are all potential symptoms of low blood levels of L-tyrosine. Many people over the age of 24 struggle with lower levels of tyrosine as a result of poor quality protein choices and protein absorption problems due to a compromised digestive system.

When suffering with mood disorders or very low energy levels, take L-tyrosine and iodine drops three times a day. Sometimes the vitamins B6, B9 (folate) and copper may be needed for those who have difficulty converting tyrosine into brain chemicals.

Suggested dosage: 500 mg 3 times per day.

Iodine
Related to L-Tyrosine and synonymous with thyroid health, iodine figures prominently in our different stages of growth and is important for many bodily functions. The thyroid gland requires a small amount of iodine daily to make thyroid hormone. It follows, then, that you should avoid iodine when the thyroid gland has become overactive or inflamed until the condition is rectified. However, depending on the iodine source and dosage, a more modest amount has shown to be helpful in certain instances of thyroid overactivity. (For a safe form of iodine when treating a hyper state, choose the homeopathic fucus.)

While commercial salt has been iodized since the 1950s, salt is an inadequate method of getting iodine into your system. Not only that, but our soil has far fewer nutrients than in years prior. In other words, a supplement is required to feed our gland's need for iodine. The good news is that iodine is an inexpensive product to buy, and there are several natural sources, such as sea plants (like kelp, dulse, and seaweed) as well as convenient liquid iodine drops. Other choices include potassium iodide, full thyroid support in a combination product, and homeopathic preparations. These should be taken daily, as directed by product of choice.[7,8,9]

Iodine is water-soluble, which means that it cannot be absorbed into tissues and held there (like our fat-soluble vitamins, A, D, E, and K2). The FDA recommends 130 mg of iodine for safety purposes, and suggests this amount of iodine can serve as protection against thyroid cancer due to radiation poisoning (even though the RDA is much lower, at 150 mcg). In fact, iodine has shown to be the only trace element that can be safely ingested in amounts up to 100,000 times that of the RDA.[10]

Testing for Thyroid Conditions

Lab tests do not always tell the whole story. The traditional thyroid tests performed at a doctor's office often show results that don't match the patient's symptoms, and even when the traditional thyroid test does show an imbalance, it is not uncommon for your thyroid gland to have been suffering for years undetected. The Thyroid Stimulating Hormone Test (TSH) is a routine blood test done to check how well your thyroid gland is functioning. Unfortunately, blood tests are not always conclusive, and the TSH is a prime example of an inaccurate test.[11,12]

For extensive information about the problems of thyroid tests performed at the doctor's office and in-depth information of thyroid health and disease reversal, please see *Reverse Thyroid Disease Naturally*.

Supporting the Adrenal Glands

As more information on our physiology is revealed, we've come to understand the impact our adrenal glands have on our thyroid when they become low functioning and imbalanced in their hormone secretions. This section will shed some light on the important role the adrenals play, and how to best nutritionally support these overachieving glands.

There are many reasons why adrenal stress reduces the conversion of certain key hormones, and why weak adrenals can cause hypothyroid symptoms, even when the thyroid does not show any deficiencies itself. One example involves adrenal stress disrupting the hypothalamic, pituitary, and adrenal axis (HPA). Chronic stress has also been shown to depress hypothalamic and pituitary function. Since these two organs direct thyroid function, any interruption of the HPA axis will also suppress thyroid function.

In other words, adrenal function must be established and adequately supported before the thyroid gland can function properly. This is because hormones secreted by the adrenal glands play crucial roles throughout the body, some of which are directly related to thyroid health and gonads.

Sources of stress to the adrenal glands include internal imbalances, such as gut inflammation and digestion problems, and a weak immune system. Other factors to consider include constant emotional stressors, such as the chronic threat of loss (of a job, financial security, or a loved one) and persistent day-to-day occurrences that ultimately deplete our body's resources.[13]

Adrenal Exhaustion and Fatigue

Symptoms of adrenal exhaustion are extreme fatigue, often accompanied by psychological stress. Unfortunately, the symptom of fatigue is not relieved by sleep. But being overtired or weak are not the worst symptoms associated with adrenal fatigue: feelings of being overwhelmed, coupled with the emotion of sadness and depression, add to an already weakened state. All too often, people suffering from adrenal fatigue or exhaustion routinely turn to stimulants like coffee and sugary beverages to get them through the day. However, their stress may also be compounded by and related to this frequent use of caffeine, alcohol, nicotine, and medications.

Under these circumstances, a person will not experience much enjoyment or happiness in their life. Other symptoms of low adrenals include higher-than-normal levels of cortisol (a stress hormone), which often signals fat storage. During this time, adrenaline may be over-produced, creating more unwanted feelings. Overproduction of unwelcome substances like cortisol and other hormones needlessly overworks the glands, weakening them. This scenario can create sugar cravings and eating binges.[14]

Diet and Supplement Suggestions for the Adrenal Glands
A broad range of vitamins and minerals should be considered when supporting the adrenal glands. Adequate nutrition through diet and supplements will lower cortisol output while aiding and relieving stress (while also reducing cravings).[15]

Many symptoms of adrenal exhaustion may be related to a deficient dietary intake of pantothenic acid, since these glands are dependent on this nutrient. B5 (pantothenic acid) is earmarked for the adrenal glands by the body, and should be balanced with the other B vitamins when taking a higher dosage of B5. Adaptogenic herbs, like ginseng and ashwagandha, are very supportive, and rhodiola and phosphatidylserine are particularly helpful. Essential fatty acids (EFAs) are highly endorsed, as with all glandular tissue issues. Glands in general want high quality protein and fats, and essential fatty acids (EFAs) are a type of good fat that the body requires for proper functioning and restoring. EFAs are always earmarked for the endocrine system as a whole and each gland or organ individually.

Avoid stimulants such as caffeine, alcohol, tobacco, soda, sugar and excessive carbohydrates, instead consume more raw vegetable juice. A few other supplements to consider include vitamins C, E, and all B vitamins, magnesium (alone or coupled with calcium), and zinc (with 2 mg of copper), bee pollen and propolis, algae (blue-green and chlorella), amino acid complex, pregnenolone and DHEA and L-Tyrosine.[16]

CONCLUSION

"PLAGUE" IS NOT a word that immediately comes to mind in today's world of modern scientific advancements. And yet that is exactly what societies worldwide are dealing with, in the form of an epidemic of depression and mood disorders. With 1.7 billion worldwide suffering from mental illness, far too many of whom go without mental health treatment, we are facing a health crisis that is all the more dangerous for how often it goes overlooked.

One need only look at the alarming statistics of depressive disorders to understand the great necessity for a prevention and treatment protocol that will not further burden the individual, their families or our health care system. That has been the main reason for the composition of this book: that the current traditional medical treatment plans we rely on are flawed.

Initial and primary care in the form of antidepressants—serotonin reuptake inhibitors and antipsychotic drugs that are not only addictive, but show diminishing returns over time—are completely inadequate to the current need. This method of treatment has raised serious concerns, with symptom outcomes shown to be far less than favorable. Scientific studies and patient reports have revealed a trail of worsening symptoms, devastation of lives and families, and violent acts upon society, all as a result of antidepressants and psychotic medications.

These issues are not going to improve with time—they will only get worse. The world as a whole must be more informed of the issues they are facing—and what is and isn't being done to address them. This book has expanded on the problems of current medications for this purpose, to help you understand this process and better protect yourself against misinformation.

The information in this book is intended to help you embrace the whole-body approach to health care, and recognize that all aspects of depressive disorders, from light mood problems to severe conditions of bipolar and schizophrenia, can be improved using a comprehensive treatment method. My goal for this book is to offer encouragement and guidance on the path to reclaiming your health. You deserve to experience life to the fullest, enjoying it with good health and a positive outlook. And with proper physical and mental self-care, you can!

PATIENT TESTIMONIALS AND CASE HISTORIES

Testimonial: Nora

Weight Loss Program, 20 Years of Antidepressant Use

I originally sought out Dr. Honda to help lose unwanted pounds. Her weight loss program was very different than what I had known in past experience—much more information on what to do with food and other body systems, etc. Dr. Honda explained the reasons why I was having difficulty controlling my appetite, and how my other issues played a role in my health as a whole, as well as my excess weight.

I started by taking six different supplements, plus Dr. Honda's juicing program. She explained in great detail why I needed the items being suggested to me, and also that some supplements are always needed in order for our bodies to support us and function optimally. She told me how there are many necessary elements that are missing in our food, because of the way our food is grown. I was never taught by any medical person what I should be eating to prevent disease and be healthy.

My energy and general health picked up quickly, but I would still have the odd eating binge and craving. The way I described my bouts of uncontrolled eating did not seem normal to Dr. Honda; she felt my long term usage of antidepressants had affected my brain chemistry, and so put together a program for me to wean off of them. I had been on Effexor and was then currently on Pristiq; she had mentioned in the beginning that this was something she wanted to work on with me, but that we first had to build up several areas of my body, such as more energy, stronger immune system, and resolving my current gut issues before we did so.

At this point in time I was feeling good, and I knew that I didn't have anything to be upset over. The new program for getting off my meds wasn't difficult; with a couple of extra supplements for the short term, I was able to easily reduce and stop my meds for the first time in 20 years. I had tried on my own several times, but within a short period of time I was able to reduce my intake. Dr. Honda explained that there are natural alternatives to most meds, since medications come from a natural source to begin with. I was given a tincture type herbal remedy that I could take whenever I felt I needed and which was non-addicting. I actually didn't need it very much!

Dr. Honda talks about empowering the body to heal while simultaneously preventing it from breaking down. I believe that the largest part of my success had to do with correcting the biochemical deficiencies in my body (as she put it), and some of the natural supplements that raised the dopamine levels in my brain. It has been months now since I have seen Dr. Honda and I am doing great and have never looked back. I realize how important it is to feel and be yourself.

Thanks Dr. Honda,

Nora

Case History: Depression/Anxiety

Subject: Male (mid-fifties), Insulin Type 2 diabetic, High blood pressure

Patient Profile

This patient was slightly similar to Nora, whose testimonial is included in the previous section. The patient's main reason for seeing me was weight loss. The weight loss program extended over a 12-week period, with check-in visits once per week. People are so often unaware of the impact their cumulative health issues have when trying to lose weight, especially when there are several drugs involved. Medications interfere with our normal biological systems; they also leech nutrients from our bodies. Adding to this scenario are the many missing key elements/nutrients necessary for repair and function, all of which make it much harder for anyone to lose the unwanted pounds that have accumulated over time.

In order for this person to lose weight, his body systems needed to be brought back to a healthy normal, which amounts to eventually reversing his diabetic condition, removing the need for antidepressants and blood pressure medication. The patient's job was demanding, as he held a senior position in a large company, and his stress levels were causing emotional eating.

Note that when the body is suffering with long-term deficiencies, our coping skills are very low, as are our metabolism and all other body functions. In such times, people visit their doctors for help and in hope of gaining an understanding for why they feel the way they do. The ultimate result is a prescription in hand, without primary imbalances being taken care of.

Patient's Main Challenge

Of all his medications and aliments, the antidepressants (Effexor and Zoloft) presented the most challenge. These drugs directly affect brain signaling and chemistry and are addictive, a dependency which worsens the longer someone remains on these types of substances.

All aspects of a patient's health must be addressed simultaneously, unless symptoms delay the employment of certain foods and substances (due to digestion and absorption problems). With this patient, we moved forward immediately.

Initial Start

Diet. Removal of all unhealthy foods at home like sugar, white flour products, white potatoes, processed or fast food, soda, alcohol, candy, ice cream, and bad fats (unhealthy cooking oils). No deep-fried food at restaurants, as well as no cold cuts or junk food.

More fresh fruits and vegetables are added. I normally add my vegetable juice formula to a patient's dietary plan, but in cases of diabetes it is delayed until sugar levels reach normal range. Considering the acid/alkaline balance of our blood matrix (20 percent acid and 80 percent alkaline), means most of what we eat in a day should consist of alkaline fruits and vegetables, while only 20 percent should consist of protein/dairy/starches.

Metabolism support. Key thyroid nutrients were added, with iodine and L-Tyrosine each taken three times per day. Other nutrients for full thyroid and body support that were missing in the greatest amounts included: omega-3 fatty acids derived from fish oil, magnesium, zinc, probiotics, B vitamins, another B and protein source called nutritional flaked yeast, as well as chromium, selenium and vitamin E.

Diabetes program. Herbal and whole, fresh foods were used to reduce and eliminate the patient's need for insulin, ultimately reversing his diabetic condition. Examples of substances used include: freshly made bitter melon juice twice a day; the herb gymnema sylvestre, taken twice a day; and a supplement carb blocker when eating more fruit or allowed starches.

While in my care, the patient was able to stop taking insulin and then continued to reduce his diabetic medication, Metformin, ultimately reversing his diabetic condition. This was very helpful in his immediate and long-term weight loss goal.

Antidepressant medication. Supporting the thyroid, adrenals and nervous/brain system, along with replacing key nutrients, creates a base of support for the systematic removal of mood enhancing or chemical balancing drugs. To bridge the gap while weaning him off of his medications and to also provide a sense of security, the patient was given a quality herbal tincture that he could use as needed: in this case, a blend of Passionflower species in a tincture preparation as well as skullcap, in the same form. These can be used together or individually for bouts of anxiety or as a sleep aid.

Because the patient's body was now being boosted on a number of levels through a whole body health approach, it was much easier for him to remove the antidepressant from his regimen.

Adrenals. Due to the patient's long-term use of antidepressant medication and complete lack of thyroid support and other necessary key nutrients, the adrenals needed attention to aid the recovery of his thyroid and boost several key hormones. In this instance, we used a quality combination product called adrenal restore *rather* than an adrenal calm product, to be taken as directed twice a day.

High blood pressure. We did not need to employ much in the way of replacing the patient's blood pressure medication. Generally, losing weight and increasing circulation lowers blood pressure. Often times, coupled with blood pressure medication is one that also works as a diuretic, which was the case with this patient. We did not need to replace the action of this drug; the additional help came from magnesium taken three times per day and a small amount of quality Hawthorn herbal tincture, taken twice a day (20 drops). After the second bottle of tincture, there was no need for repeated doses. These by themselves would not have worked as well if the body had not been more fully supported.

Initial Results

The patient was very happy with the program and its results. He lost his desired weight, which in his (and my) opinion was second in achievement to reversing his other deteriorating health issues. He no longer requires medications for diabetes, blood pressure or antidepressants.

Post-Program Report

Many months after the completion of this program, the patient met someone at work who hadn't seen him in a long while and remarked how different he seemed to be. This was more than just his weight loss; it was a remark on his general responses and interactions with others.

Here is the point I wish to make from this case. Some people on antidepressant medication do not realize how they appear to others they interact with. Certainly, they can appear as they would normally, but more often, there are either subtle or obvious character/personality changes occurring: a more rapid way of speaking and anxiousness; it becomes hard for them to focus and concentrate on what is being said to them; their minds seem to be racing; they are more timid and withdrawn.

Bad habits increase and sometimes take over the lives of these individuals. As their condition progresses into a chronic mood disorder, they lose their jobs, lose interest in hobbies and other activities that were main features of their lives. Insecurity is often part of this scenario, and presents with both mood disorders and mental illness alike.

Major life changes occur and most often continue to do so; but when a person becomes severally altered by psychotic drugs, they are no longer able to make decisions, live life normally or care for themselves properly.

ABOUT THE AUTHOR

MICHELLE HONDA, PH.D. is a holistic doctor who specializes in disease reversal through the employment of natural medicine and clinical nutrition. Within two years of finishing her Ph.D., Michelle opened a Holistic Health Clinic with her husband Ron Honda, called Renew You Holistic Health (www.renewyou.ca) in Ancaster, Ontario, Canada. She now resides in Guysborough, Nova Scotia, Canada, where she conducts her private practice.

Author of the innovative book *Reverse Gut Disease Naturally*, Michelle is wholly devoted to the welfare of mankind and the preservation of the environment. Her success in full disease reversal of intestinal complaints is unprecedented, and she has developed a reputation for being an expert in the field of applied natural medicine and clinical nutrition.

Michelle has applied this same expertise to every book in her series of natural health books, including *Reverse Heart Disease Naturally*, *Reverse Inflammation Naturally*, *Reverse Thyroid Disease Naturally* and *Reverse Alzheimer's Disease Naturally*. Michelle is passionate about sharing knowledge and offering readers the power of personal choice, enabling them to restore, renew and rejuvenate themselves. To this end, Michelle continues to publish informative articles enlightening others on their journey to wellness.

Visit Michelle Honda at her website: www.michellehonda.com

BIBLIOGRAPHY

Introduction

1. Mental Myths and Facts. (2017). https://www.mentalhealth.gov/basics/mental-health-myths-facts

2. Depression and Other Common Mental Disorders: Global Health Estimates. Geneva: World Health Organization. 2017. http://apps.who.int/iris/bitstream/10665/254610/1/WHO-MSD-MER-2017.2-eng.pdf

3. Crutin. Increase in suicide in the United States. 1999-2014. NCHS data brief.no 241. https://www.cdc.gov/nchs/products/databriefs/db241.htm

Chapter 1

1. Any Mental Illness (AMI) Among Adults. (n.d.). Retrieved October 23, 2015, from http://www.nimh.nih.gov/health/statistics/prevalence/any-mental-illness-ami-among-adults.shtml

2. Serious Mental Illness (SMI) Among Adults. (n.d.). Retrieved October 23, 2015, from http://www.nimh.nih.gov/health/statistics/prevalence/serious-mental-illness-smi-among-us-adults.shtml

3. Any Disorder Among Children. (n.d.) Retrieved January 16, 2015, from http://www.nimh.nih.gov/health/statistics/prevalence/any-disorder-among-children.shtml

4. Schizophrenia. (n.d.). Retrieved January 16, 2015, from http://www.nimh.nih.gov/health/statistics/prevalence/schizophrenia.shtml

5. Bipolar Disorder Among Adults. (n.d.). Retrieved January 16, 2015, from http://www.nimh.nih.gov/health/statistics/prevalence/bipolar-disorder-among-adults.shtml

6. Any Anxiety Disorder Among Adults. (n.d.). Retrieved January 16, 2015, from http://www.nimh.nih.gov/health/statistics/prevalence/any-anxiety-disorder-among-adults.shtml

7. Substance Abuse and Mental Health Services Administration, Results from the 2014 National Survey on Drug Use and Health: Mental Health Findings, NSDUH Series H-50, HHS Publication No. (SMA) 15-4927. Rockville, MD: Substance Abuse and Mental Health Services Administration. (2015). Retrieved October 27, 2015 from http://www.

samhsa.gov/data/sites/default/files/NSDUH-FRR1-2014/NSDUH-FRR1-2014.pdf

8.   Tracey Watson. World famous psychiatrist warns that increased use of psychiatric drugs will translate to more mass shootings. March 21, 2018. http://www.wakingtimes.com/2018/02/27/world-famous-psychiatrist-says-psychiatric-drug-treatment-means-mass-shootings-will-happen/

9.   Watson, N.V., & Breedlove, S.M. (2012). The mind's machine. Foundations of brain and behavior. Sunderland, Massachussets, USA: Sinauer Associates, Inc. Publishers. https://www.amazon.ca/Minds-Machine-Foundations-Brain-Behavior/dp/0878939334

10. Grader, E., & Bateman, A. (2017). Introduction to brain anatomy and mechanisms of injury. In R. Winson, B.A. Wilson, & A. Bateman (Eds.), The brain injury rehabilitation workbook. (pp. 15-35). New York: Guilford Press. https://www.guilford.com/books/The-Brain-Injury-Rehabilitation-Workbook/Winson-Wilson-Bateman/9781462528509

11. Higging, E.S., & George, M.S. (2009). Brain stimulation therapies for clinicians. Washington DC: American Psychiatric Publishing, Inc. https://www.appi.org/Brain_Stimulation_Therapies_for_Clinicians

12. Zimmermann, M. (2001). Burgerstein's handbook of nutrition. Micronutrients in the prevention and therapy of disease. New York: Thieme. http://197.14.51.10:81/pmb/AGROALIMENTAIRE/Handbook%20of%20Nutrition.pdf

13. Mozaffarian, D. (2012). The truth about vitamins and minerals. Choosing the nutrients you need to stay healthy. Boston, USA: Harvard Health Publications. https://blog.content.health.harvard.edu/blog/special-reports/the-truth-about-vitamins-and-minerals-choosing-the-nutrients-you-need-to-stay-healthy

14. Kaplan, B. J., & Leung, B. (2011). Micronutrient treatment of mental disorders. Integrative Medicine: A Clinician's Journal, 10(3), 32-39. https://www.researchgate.net/publication/230800944_Micronutrient_treatment_of_mental_disorders

15. Siever, L.J. (2008). Neurobiology of aggression and violence. American Journal of Psychiatry 165, 429–442. https://ajp.psychiatryonline.org/doi/abs/10.1176/appi.ajp.2008.07111774

16. Zaalberg, A., Nijman, H., Bulten, E., Stroosma, L., & van der Staak, C. (2009). Effects of nutritional supplements on aggression, rule-breaking, and psychopathology among young adult prisoners. Aggressive Behavior, 35, 1–10. https://www.ncbi.nlm.nih.gov/pubmed/20014286

Chapter 2

1. Noury J.L., Nardo J.M., Healy D., Jureidini J., Raven M., Tufanaru C. & Abi-Jaoude E. (2015) Restoring Study 329: efficacy and harms of paroxetine and imipramine in treatment of major depression in adolescence. BMJ 351, h4320. doi:10.1136/bmj.h4320. https://www.ncbi.nlm.nih.gov/pubmed/26376805

2. Orthomolecular Applications in Integrative Psychiatry – Biological Models for Suicide Prevention. Online Course presented by James Greenblatt, MD. March, 2019. https://isom.ca/event/suicide-prevention/

3. Paul W. Andrews, Lyndsey Gott & J. Anderson Thomson, Jr. Things Your Doctor Should Tell You About Antidepressants. February 19, 2018. https://www.madinamerica.com/2012/09/things-your-doctor-should-tell-you-about-antidepressants/

4. Front. Psychol., 24 April 2012 | https://doi.org/10.3389/fpsyg.2012.00117. Primum non nocere: an evolutionary analysis of whether antidepressants do more harm than good. https://www.frontiersin.org/articles/10.3389/fpsyg.2012.00117/full

5. Berger, M., Gray, J. A., and Roth, B. L. (2009). The expanded biology of serotonin. Annu. Rev. Med. 60, 355–366. https://www.ncbi.nlm.nih.gov/pmc/articles/PMC5864293/

6. Kirsch, I., Deacon, B. J., Huedo-Medina, T. B., Scoboria, A., Moore, T. J., and Johnson, B. T. (2008). Initial severity and antidepressant benefits: a meta-analysis of data submitted to the food and drug administration. PloS Med. 5, e45. doi:10.1371/journal.pmed.0050045. https://www.ncbi.nlm.nih.gov/pubmed/18303940

7. Bonin, R. (2012). "Treating depression: is there a placebo effect?" in 60 Minutes (New York, NY: CBS Broadcasting, Inc.). https://www.cbsnews.com/news/treating-depression-is-there-a-placebo-effect/

8. Khan, A., Brodhead, A. E., Kolts, R. L., and Brown, W. A. (2005). Severity of depressive symptoms and response to antidepressants and placebo in antidepressant trials. J. Psychiatr. Res. 39, 145–150. https://www.ncbi.nlm.nih.gov/pubmed/15589562

9. Rutter, J. J., and Auerbach, S. B. (1993). Acute uptake inhibition increases extracellular serotonin in the rat forebrain. J. Pharmacol. Exp. Ther. 265, 1319–1324. https://www.ncbi.nlm.nih.gov/pubmed/7685386

10. Best, J., Nijhout, H. F., and Reed, M. (2010). Serotonin synthesis, release and reuptake in terminals: a mathematical model. Theor. Biol. Med. Model. 7. doi: 10.1186/1742-4682-7-34 https://www.ncbi.nlm.nih.gov/pubmed/20723248

11. Honig, G., Jongsma, M. E., van der Hart, M. C. G., and Tecott, L. H. (2009). Chronic citalopram administration causes a sustained suppression of serotonin synthesis in the mouse forebrain. PLoS ONE 4, e6797. doi:10.1371/journal.pone.0006797. https://www.ncbi.nlm.nih.gov/pmc/articles/PMC2728775/

12. Bartholoma, P., Erlandsson, N., Kaufmann, K., Rossler, O. G., Baumann, B., Wirth, T., Giehl, K. M., and Thiel, G. (2002). Neuronal cell death induced by antidepressants: lack of correlation with Egr-1, NF-kappa B and extracellular signal-regulated protein kinase activation. Biochem. Pharmacol. 63, 1507–1516. https://www.ncbi.nlm.nih.gov/pubmed/11996893

13. Post, A., Crochemore, C., Uhr, M., Holsboer, F., and Behl, C. (2000). Differential effects of antidepressants on the viability of clonal hippocampal cells. Biol. Psychiatry 47, 138. https://www.biologicalpsychiatryjournal.com/article/S0006-3223(00)00721-6/abstract?mobileUi=0

14. Sairanen, M., Lucas, G., Ernfors, P., Castren, M., and Castren, E. (2005). Brain-derived neurotrophic factor and antidepressant drugs have different but coordinated effects on neuronal turnover, proliferation, and survival in the adult dentate gyrus. J. Neurosci. 25, 1089–1094. https://www.ncbi.nlm.nih.gov/pubmed/15689544

15. Rutter, J. J., and Auerbach, S. B. (1993). Acute uptake inhibition increases extracellular serotonin in the rat forebrain. J. Pharmacol. Exp. Ther. 265, 1319–1324. https://www.ncbi.nlm.nih.gov/pubmed/7685386

16. Krämer, U.M., Riba, J., Ritcher, S., & Münte, T.F. (2011). An fMRI study on the role of serotonin in reactive aggression. PLoS ONE, 6(11), 1-8. http://journals.plos.org/plosone/article?id=10.1371/journal.pone.0027668

17. Krug, E., et al., (2002). World Report on Violence and Health. Geneva: World Health Organization. http://www.who.int/violence_injury_prevention/violence/world_report/en/introduction.pdf

18. Federal Investigation into Link Between Psych Drugs and School Shootings. Constitutional Attorney Jonathan Emord. By J. D. Heyes and Atty. Jonathan Emord.Global Research, February 22, 2018. NaturalNews.com 21 February 2018.https://www.globalresearch.ca/federal-investigation-into-link-between-psych-drugs-and-school-shootings/5629959

19. Mercadillo, R.E., & Arias, N.A. (2011). Violence and compassion: a bioethical insight into their cognitive bases and social manifestations. International Social Science Journal 221-232. https://www.ncbi.nlm.nih.gov/pmc/articles/PMC4334407/

20. McCabe, P.C., & Shaw, .S.R. (2010). Developments in neuropsychiatric treatment. In. McCabe, P.C., & Shaw, S.R. (Eds.), Psychiatric disorders. Current topics and interventions for education. (pp. 2-7). California, USA: National Association of School Psychologists & CORWIN. https://www.isom.ca/wp-content/uploads/2017/10/Nutrient-Depletion-Induced-Neuro-Chemical-Disorder-Brain-Hunger-as-the-Basis-of-Psychopathology-and-Aggressive-Behavior-32.5.pdf

21. Pliszka, S.R. (2016). Neuroscience for the mental health clinician. (2nd ed). New York: The Guilford Press. https://www.guilford.com/books/Neuroscience-for-the-Mental-Health-Clinician/Steven-Pliszka/9781462527113

22. José R. Rodríguez, Michael J. González, Jorge Miranda.Nutritional deficiencies and maladaptive behaviors: a possible new paradigm for the prevention of aggressive behaviors. Vol 18, No 2 (2008). http://revistas.uv.mx/index.php/psicysalud/article/view/662

23. Davidson, K.M., & Kaplan, B.J. (2012). Nutrient intakes are correlated with overall psychiatric functioning in adults with mood disorders. The Canadian Journal of Psychiatry, 57(2), 85-92. https://www.ncbi.nlm.nih.gov/pubmed/22340148

24. Zaalberg, A., Nijman, H., Bulten, E., Stroosma, L., & van der Staak, C. (2009). Effects of nutritional supplements on aggression, rule-breaking, and psychopathology among young adult prisoners. Aggressive Behavior, 35, 1–10. https://www.ncbi.nlm.nih.gov/pubmed/20014286

Chapter 3

1. What is serotonin simple definition? https://simple.wikipedia.org/wiki/Serotonin

2. Serotonin: Facts, uses, SSRIs, and sources - Medical News Today. https://www.medicalnewstoday.com/kc/serotonin-facts-232248

3. Oct 12, 2011Serotonin and Depression: 9 Questions and Answers – WebMD. https://www.webmd.com/depression/features/serotonin

4. Serotonin and Serotonin Deficiency - Integrative Psychiatry. https://www.integrativepsychiatry.net/seritonin-and-seritonin-deficiency.html

5. Serotonin - Integrative Psychiatry. https://www.integrativepsychiatry.net/serotonin.html

6. New Blood and Urine Tests Find 5 Distinct Types of Depression. https://www.healthline.com/health.../researcher-identifies-five-types-of-depression-0508

7.   New Blood and Urine Tests Find 5 Distinct Types of Depression. https://www.healthline.com/health.../researcher-identifies-five-types-of-depression-0508

8.   New Blood and Urine Tests Find 5 Distinct Types of Depression, Researcher Says. https://www.healthline.com/health-news/researcher-identifies-five-types-of-depression-050814#1

9.   Neumeister A. Tryptophan depletion, serotonin, and depression: where do we stand? Psychopharmacology Bulletin [01 Jan 2003, 37(4):99-115]. http://europepmc.org/abstract/MED/15131521

10.   V Maletic,1 M Robinson,2 T Oakes,2 S Iyengar,2 S G Ball,2,3 and J Russell2. Neurobiology of depression: an integrated view of key findings. Int J Clin Pract. 2007 Dec; 61(12): 2030–2040. https://www.ncbi.nlm.nih.gov/pmc/articles/PMC2228409/

11.   Riedel WJ1, Klaassen T, Schmitt JA. Tryptophan, mood, and cognitive function. Brain Behav Immun. 2002 Oct;16(5):581-9. https://www.ncbi.nlm.nih.gov/pubmed/12401472

12.   Tryptophan . https://en.wikipedia.org/wiki/Tryptophan

13.   Science News: Omega-3 fatty acids, vitamin D may control brain serotonin, affecting behavior and psychiatric disorders. UCSF Benioff Children's Hospital Oakland. February 25, 2015. https://www.sciencedaily.com/releases/2015/02/150225094109.htm

14.   Katie M. Vance,1 David M. Ribnicky,2 Gerlinda E. Hermann,1 and Richard C. Rogers1. St. John's Wort enhances the synaptic activity of the nucleus of the solitary tract. Nutrition. 2014 Jul-Aug; 30(0 0): S37–S42. https://www.ncbi.nlm.nih.gov/pmc/articles/PMC4128486/

15.   FASEB J. 2015 Jun;29(6):2207-22. Vitamin D and the omega-3 fatty acids control serotonin synthesis and action, part 2: relevance for ADHD, bipolar disorder, schizophrenia, and impulsive behavior. https://www.ncbi.nlm.nih.gov/pubmed/25713056

16.   Emily K. Tarleton , Benjamin Littenberg, Charles D. MacLean, Amanda G. Kennedy, Christopher Daley. Role of magnesium supplementation in the treatment of depression. June 27, 2017. https://journals.plos.org/plosone/article?id=10.1371/journal.pone.0180067

17.   Urszula Doboszewska, 1 , 2 Piotr Wlaź, 2 Gabriel Nowak, 1 , 3 Maria Radziwoń-Zaleska, 4 Ranji Cui, 5 and Katarzyna Młyniec 1. Zinc in the Monoaminergic Theory of Depression: Its Relationship to Neural Plasticity. 2017 Feb 19. https://www.ncbi.nlm.nih.gov/pmc/articles/PMC5337390/

18. Kennedy, David O.B Vitamins and the Brain: Mechanisms, Dose and Efficacy. Journal ListNutrientsv.8(2); 2016 FebPMC4772032. https://www.ncbi.nlm.nih.gov/pmc/articles/PMC4772032/

19. Nathan PJ1, Lu K, Gray M, Oliver C. The neuropharmacology of L-theanine(N-ethyl-L-glutamine): a possible neuroprotective and cognitive enhancing agent. J Herb Pharmacother. 2006;6(2):21-30. https://www.ncbi.nlm.nih.gov/pubmed/17182482

20. S. K. Kulkarni* and A. Dhir1. An Overview of Curcumin in Neurological Disorders. Indian J Pharm Sci. 2010 Mar-Apr; 72(2): 149–154. https://www.ncbi.nlm.nih.gov/pmc/articles/PMC2929771/

Chapter 4

1.   Jeff Hayward, Uncovering 8 Signs of Perfectly Hidden Depression. http://www.activebeat.co/your-health/uncovering-8-signs-of-perfectly-hidden-depression/

2.   HuffingtonPost.com. https://www.huffingtonpost.com/entry/the-ten-traits-of-perfectly-hidden-depression_us_59133807e4b07e366cebb7e9

3.   Dr. Aaron T. Beck, The Beck Depression Inventory Test. http://treat-depression.com/depression-test

4.   Robert Lock, 7 Things People With Hidden Depression Do. https://www.lifehack.org/articles/communication/7-things-people-with-hidden-depression.html

5.   Dr. Margaret Rutherford, How to Know if You Experience Perfectly Hidden Depression. April 24, 2016. https://goodmenproject.com/featured-content/know-experience-perfectly-hidden-depression-kt/

6.   M. Honda PhD. Reverse Gut Diseases Naturally, 2015. http://michelle-honda-blog.renewyou.ca/crohns-colitis-book/

7.   M. Honda PhD. Reverse Thyroid Disease Naturally. 2018. http://michelle-honda-blog.renewyou.ca/reverse-thyroid-disease-naturally/

8.   R H Yolken and E F Torrey, Clin Microbiol Rev. 1995 Jan; 8(1): 131–145. Viruses, schizophrenia, and bipolar disorder. https://www.ncbi.nlm.nih.gov/pmc/articles/PMC172852/

9.   American Psychiatrie Association. Diagnostic and Statistical Manual of Mental Disorders. Fourth Edition. Washington, DC: American Psychiatric Association; 1994. https://justines2010blog.files.wordpress.com/2011/03/dsm-iv.pdf

10. National Institute of Mental Health Anxiety Disorders Research at the National Institute of Mental Health, December 7, 2002. Accessed 02, 26, 2018. https://www.nimh.nih.gov/index.shtml

11. Kessler RC., Wittchen HU. Patterns and correlates of generalized anxiety disorder in community samples. J Clin Psychiatry. 2002;63(suppl 8):4–10. https://www.ncbi.nlm.nih.gov/pubmed/12044107

12. Gorman JM. Treatment of generalized anxiety disorder. J Clin Psychiatry. 2002;63(suppl8):17–23. https://www.ncbi.nlm.nih.gov/pubmed/12044104

13. Masand PS., Gupta S. Selective serotonin-reuptake inhibitors: an update. Harv Rev Psychiatry. 1999;7:69–84. https://www.ncbi.nlm.nih.gov/pubmed/10471245

14. Barbey JT., Roose SP. SSRI safety in overdose. J Clin Psychiatry. 1998;59(suppl 15):42–48. https://www.ncbi.nlm.nih.gov/pubmed/9786310

15. Lisa L. von Moltke, David J. Greenblatt, MD, D. Medication dependence and anxiety. Department of Pharmacology and Experimental Therapeutics, Tufts University School of Medicine and Tufts-New England Medical Center, Boston, Mass, USA; Dialogues Clin Neurosci. 2003 Sep; 5(3): 237–245. https://www.ncbi.nlm.nih.gov/pmc/articles/PMC3181633/

16. Brauer HR., Nowicki PW., Catalane G., Catalane MC. Panic attacks associated with citalopram. South Medj. 2002;95:1088–1089. https://www.ncbi.nlm.nih.gov/pmc/articles/PMC3181633/

17. Catalano G., Hakala SM., Catalane MC. Sertraline-induced panic attacks. Clin Neuropharmacol. 2000;23:164–168. https://www.ncbi.nlm.nih.gov/pmc/articles/PMC3181633/

18. Greenblatt DJ., von Moltke LL., Harmatz JS., Shader Rl. Human cytochromes and some newer antidepressants: kinetics, metabolism, and drug interactions. J Clin Psychopharrnacol. 1999;19(5 suppl 1):23S–35S. http://journals.sagepub.com/doi/abs/10.1177/089719001129040964

19. Posternak MA., Mueller Tl. Assessing the risks and benefits of benzodiazepines for anxiety disorders in patients with a history of substance abuse or dependence. Am J Addict. 2001;10:48–68. https://www.ncbi.nlm.nih.gov/pubmed/11268828

20. Kandel DB., Huang FY., Davies M. Comorbidity between patterns of substance use dependence and psychiatric syndromes. Drug Alcohol Depend. 2001;64:233–241. https://www.ncbi.nlm.nih.gov/pmc/articles/PMC2653612/

21. Conway KP., Swendsen JD., Rounsaville BJ., Merikangas KR. Personality, drug of choice, and comorbid psychopathology among substance abusers. Drug Alcohol Depend. 2002;65:225–234. https://www.ncbi.nlm.nih.

gov/pubmed/11841894 - 2001;36:219–223. https://academic.oup.com/alcalc/article/36/3/219/170138

22. Kan CC., Breteler MH., van der Ven AH., et al. Assessment of benzodiazepine dependence in alcohol and drug dependent outpatients: a research report. Subst Use Misuse. 2001;36:1085–1096. http://www.tandfonline.com/doi/abs/10.1081/JA-100104491

23. Becona E., Vazquez FL., Miguez MC. Smoking cessation and anxiety in a clinical sample. Personality individual Differences. 2002;32:489–494. https://www.ncbi.nlm.nih.gov/pmc/articles/PMC4122254/

24. Schuckit MA., Hesselbrock V. Alcohol dependence and anxiety disorders: what is the relationship?. Am J Psychiatry. 1994;151:1723–34. https://www.ncbi.nlm.nih.gov/pubmed/7977877

25. 25.Kushner MG. Relationship between alcohol problems and anxiety disorders. Am J Psychiatry. 1996;153:139–140. https://ajp.psychiatryonline.org/doi/ref/10.1176/ajp.156.5.723

26. Westra HA., Stewart SH. As-needed use of benzodiazepines in managing clinical anxiety: incidence and implications. Curr Pharm Design. 2002;8:59–74. https://www.ncbi.nlm.nih.gov/pubmed/11812250

27. Farrell M., Howes S., Taylor C., et al. Substance misuse and psychiatric comorbidity: an overview of the OPCS National Psychiatric Morbidity Survey. Addict Behav. 1998;23:909–918. https://www.ncbi.nlm.nih.gov/pubmed/9801725

28. Bipolar Disorder vs. Depression: What's the Difference? - WebMD. https://www.webmd.com/bipolar-disorder/bipolar-vs-depression

29. Bipolar and Depression - Bipolar Disorder Center - EverydayHealth. https://www.everydayhealth.com/bipolar-disorder/bipolar-disorder-and-depression.aspx

30. Medical Definition of Hypomania. https://www.medicinenet.com/script/main/art.asp?articlekey=30745

31. Is anger a symptom of bipolar? https://www.bphope.com/stuck-on-the-rage-road/

32. What is a Major Depressive Episode? - Bridges to Recovery. https://www.bridgestorecovery.com/major-depression/what-is-a-major-depressive-episode/

33. Take Bipolar Disorder Seriously – WebMD. https://www.webmd.com/bipolar-disorder/news/.../take-bipolar-disorder-seriously

34. Does Depression Go Away on Its Own With Time? - Verywell Mind. https://www.verywellmind.com/does-depression-go-away-on-its-own-with-time-1067582

35. Donna Jackel, Everything You Ever Wanted To Know About BIPOLAR DEPRESSION. 2010. https://www.bphope.com/everything-you-ever-wanted-to-know-about-bipolar-depression/

Chapter 5

1. Schizophrenia – Fact Sheet - Treatment Advocacy Center. www.treatmentadvocacycenter.org/evidence-and.../learn.../25-schizophrenia-fact-sheet

2. A typological model of schizophrenia based on age at onset, sex and familial morbidity. Acta Psych8atr. Scand. 89, 135-141 (1994). https://www.ncbi.nlm.nih.gov/pubmed/8178665

3. Schizophrenia Facts and Statistics - Schizophrenia.com. www.schizophrenia.com/szfacts.htm

4. Neuropsychiatry Review. Cardiff University. "Genetics researchers close in on schizophrenia: 50 new gene regions that increase risk of developing schizophrenia." ScienceDaily. ScienceDaily, 27 February 2018. www.sciencedaily.com/releases/2018/02/180227111701.htm

5. What Is Paranoid Schizophrenia?https://www.webmd.com/schizophrenia/guide/schizophrenia-paranoia#1

6. Jarid Goodman1 and Mark G. Packard1. Memory Systems and the Addicted Brain. https://www.ncbi.nlm.nih.gov/pmc/articles/PMC4766276/

7. Brain Damage Caused by Neuroleptic Psychiatric Drugs — MFIPortal. www.mindfreedom.org/kb/psychiatric-drugs/antipsychotics/neuroleptic-brain-damage

Chapter 6

1. Bruce S. McEwen, Author, Elizabeth Norton Lasley, Author with Elizabeth N. Lasley. The end of stress as we know it. https://www.publishersweekly.com/978-0-309-07640-1

2. The Mind and Mental Health: How Stress Affects the Brain. https://www.tuw.edu/content/health/how-stress-affects-the-brain/

3. Brain Structure & Function. https://www.ncbi.nlm.nih.gov/pmc/articles/PMC2522333/

4. Prefrontal cortex. https://en.wikipedia.org/wiki/Prefrontal_cortex

5. Brain Structure & Function. https://www.ncbi.nlm.nih.gov/pmc/articles/PMC2522333/

6. Amygdala's Role in Emotion: Function & Overview. https://study.com/academy/lesson/amygdala-role-in-emotion-function-lesson-quiz.html

7.   Hippocampus Functions - News-Medical.Net. https://www.news-medical.net/health/Hippocampus-Functions.aspx

8.   Brain Structure & Function. https://www.ncbi.nlm.nih.gov/pmc/articles/PMC2522333/

9.   Limbic system. https://en.wikipedia.org/wiki/Limbic_system

10.   JAMA Intern Med. 2015 Mar;175(3):401-7. doi: 10.1001/jamainternmed.2014.7663. Cumulative use of strong anticholinergics and incident dementia: a prospective cohort study. Gray SL1, Anderson ML2, Dublin S3, Hanlon JT4, Hubbard R5, Walker R2, Yu O2, Crane PK6, Larson EB7. https://www.ncbi.nlm.nih.gov/pubmed/25621434

11.   Shelly Gray, PharmD, MS. Anticholinergics and Risk of Dementia, School of Pharmacy University of Washington. http://depts.washington.edu/uwconf/eff/resources/5GRAY_ACTalkEFF.pdf

12.   Daniel M I Britt1,2 and Gregory S Day, MD, MSc, FRCPC1,3. Over-Prescribed Medications, Under-Appreciated Risks: A review of the cognitive effects of anticholinergic medications in older adults. https://www.ncbi.nlm.nih.gov/pmc/articles/PMC5125613/

13.   Beverly Merz. Common anticholinergic drugs like Benadryl linked to increased dementia risk—Harvard Health Blog, Updated May 23, 2017. http://www.health.harvard.edu/blog/common-anticholinergic-drugs-like-benadryl-linked-increased-dementia-risk-201501287667

Chapter 7

1.   Postpartum depression - Symptoms and causes - Mayo Clinic. https://www.mayoclinic.org/diseases-conditions/postpartum-depression/.../syc-20376617

2.   American Pregnancy Association. http://americanpregnancy.org/first-year-of-life/baby-blues/3. Postpartum Depression and the Baby Blues: Signs, Symptoms.

3.   https://www.helpguide.org/.../depression/postpartum-depression-and-the-baby-blues.htm

4.   Genetic Predictors of Postpartum Depression Uncovered by Johns Hopkins Researchers. https://www.hopkinsmedicine.org/news/media/releases/genetic_predictors_of_postpartum_depression_uncovered_by_johns_hopkins_researchers

5.   Statistics by Country for Postpartum depression. https://www.rightdiagnosis.com/p/postpartum_depression/stats-country.htm

6.   Types of Postpartum Depression and How to Cope. Nancy Schimelpfening. November 26, 2018. https://www.verywellmind.com/postpartum-depression-types-1067039

7.   Postpartum Depression Statistics. https://www.postpartumdepression.org/resources/statistics/

8.   Understanding Postpartum Depression -- Diagnosis and Treatment. https://www.webmd.com/depression/postpartum-depression/understanding-postpartum-depression-treatment#1

9.   Postpartum Depression. Medical Author: Roxanne Dryden-Edwards, MD Medical Editor: William C. Shiel Jr., MD, FACP, FACR. http://www.medicinenet.com/postpartum_depression/page4.htm

10.   The Ammon-Pinizzotto Center for Women's Mental Health at MGH. https://womensmentalhealth.org/ and https://womensmentalhealth.org/specialty-clinics/postpartum-psychiatric-disorders/?doing_wp_cron=147 5415220.4255061149597167968750

11.   Postpartum Depression. https://adaa.org/living-with-anxiety/women/postpartum-depression

12.   Postpartum Depression Medication. https://www.postpartumdepression.org/treatment/postpartum-depression-medication/

13.   Beck Institute for Cognitive Behavior Therapy. https://beckinstitute.org/get-informed/what-is-cognitive-therapy/

14.   What Is Cognitive Behavioral Therapy? https://www.psychologytoday.com/ca/basics/cognitive-behavioral-therapy

15.   Interpersonal Psychotherapy (IPT). https://www.camh.ca/en/health-info/mental-illness-and-addiction-index/interpersonal-psychotherapy

16.   Kirsten Weir. December 2011, Vol 42, No. 11.The Exercise Effect – Benefits of exercise and why it should be used more frequently in mental health treatment. (American Psychological Association). https://www.apa.org/monitor/2011/12/exercise

17.   The Exercise Prescription for Depression, Anxiety, and Stress. Lawrence Robinson, Jeanne Segal, Ph.D., and Melinda Smith, M.A. Last updated: November 2018. https://www.helpguide.org/articles/healthy-living/the-mental-health-benefits-of-exercise.htm/

18.   Dr Piotr Wozniak, May 2012. Good sleep, good learning, good life. https://www.supermemo.com/en/articles/sleep

19.   Organclock. https://foreverconscious.com/traditional-chinese-organ-body-clock

Chapter 8

1. Which Came First, Depression or Alcoholism? - The Ranch. https://www.recoveryranch.com/articles/.../which-came-first-depression-or-alcoholism/

2. Can Alcohol Induce Depression? https://americanaddictioncenters.org/alcoholism-treatment/depression/

3. Howard J. Edenberg, Ph.D. The Genetics of Alcohol Metabolism: Role of Alcohol Dehydrogenase. https://americanaddictioncenters.org/alcoholism-treatment/depression

4. Aldehyde Dehydrogenase Variants. Alcohol Res Health. 2007; 30(1): 5–13. https://www.ncbi.nlm.nih.gov/pmc/articles/PMC3860432/

5. NIAAA Publications - National Institute on Alcohol Abuse and Alcoholism. https://pubs.niaaa.nih.gov/publications/aa72/aa72.htm

6. Howard J. Edenberg, Ph.D. The Genetics of Alcohol Metabolism: Role of Alcohol Dehydrogenase and Aldehyde Dehydrogenase Variants. Alcohol Res Health. 2007; 30(1): 5–13. https://www.ncbi.nlm.nih.gov/pmc/articles/PMC3860432/

7. Variations in ADH and ALDH in Southwest California Indians. https://pubs.niaaa.nih.gov/publications/arh301/14-17.htm

8. Alcohol Alert banner.Number 72. July 2007. Alcohol Metabolizing Process. https://pubs.niaaa.nih.gov/publications/aa72/aa72.htm

9. Alcohol and Your Body | Health Promotion | Brown University. https://www.brown.edu/campus-life/health/services/...other.../alcohol-and-your-body

10. Alcohol and Your Body - UCSC S.H.O.P Student Health Center. https://shop.ucsc.edu/alcohol-other-drugs/alcohol/your-body.html

11. NIDA. https://www.drugabuse.gov/publications/principles-drug-addiction-treatment-research-based-guide-third-edition/evidence-based-approaches-to-drug-addiction-treatment/behavioral

12. Day E, Bentham P, Callaghan R, Kuruvilla T, George S. Thiamine for Wernicke-Korsakoff Syndrome in people at risk from alcohol abuse. Cochrane Database Syst Rev. 2004. CD004033. https://www.ncbi.nlm.nih.gov/pubmed/23818100

13. MedlinePlus.Wernicke-Korsakoff syndrome. https://medlineplus.gov/ency/article/000771.htm

14. Glen L Xiong, MD; Chief Editor: David Bienenfeld, MD . Wernicke-Korsakoff Syndrome Medication.Updated: Jun 09, 2017. https://emedicine.medscape.com/article/288379-medication

15. Thomson AD, Cook CC, Touquet R, Henry JA. The Royal College of Physicians report on alcohol: guidelines for managing Wernicke's encephalopathy in the accident and Emergency Department. Alcohol. 2002 Nov-Dec. 37(6):513-21.

16. Galvin R, Bråthen G, Ivashynka A, Hillbom M, Tanasescu R, Leone MA. EFNS guidelines for diagnosis, therapy and prevention of Wernicke encephalopathy. Eur J Neurol. 2010 Dec. 17(12):1408-18. https://www.ncbi.nlm.nih.gov/pubmed/20642790

17. Isenberg-Grzeda E, Kutner HE, Nicolson SE. Wernicke-Korsakoff-syndrome: under-recognized and under-treated. Psychosomatics. 2012 Nov-Dec. 53(6):507-16. https://www.ncbi.nlm.nih.gov/pubmed/23157990

18. Home Remedies, Herbs, and Food Supplements for Wernicke-Korsakoff Syndrome. https://www.curesdecoded.com/conditions/wernicke-korsakoff-syndrome/335

Chapter 9
1. Annie Shirwaikar, Raghavan Govindarajan, Ajay Kumar Singh Rawat. Integrating Complementary and Alternative Medicine with Primary Health Care. Evid Based Complement Alternat Med. 2013; 2013: 948308. https://www.ncbi.nlm.nih.gov/pmc/articles/PMC3728503/

2. Ernst E, Resch KL, Mills S, et al. Complementary medicine—a definition. British Journal of General Practice. 1995;45(article 506) https://www.ncbi.nlm.nih.gov/pmc/articles/PMC1239386/

3. Barnes J, Abbot NC, Harkness EF, Ernst E. Articles on complementary medicine in the mainstream medical literature: an investigation of MEDLINE, 1966 through 1996. Arch Intern Med. 1999 Aug 9-23; 159(15):1721-5. https://www.ncbi.nlm.nih.gov/pubmed/10448774

4. Brevoort P. The booming US botanical market: a new overview. Herbal Gram. 1998;44:33–48. https://eurekamag.com/research/003/297/003297973.php

5. Unconventional medicine in the United States. Prevalence, costs, and patterns of use. Eisenberg DM, Kessler RC, Foster C, Norlock FE, Calkins DR, Delbanco TLN Engl J Med. 1993 Jan 28; 328(4):246-52. https://www.ncbi.nlm.nih.gov/pubmed/8418405

6. Pelletier KR, Marie A, Krasner M, Haskell WL. Review Current trends in the integration and reimbursement of complementary and alternative medicine by managed care, insurance carriers, and hospital providers. Am J Health Promot. 1997 Nov-Dec; 12(2):112-22. https://www.ncbi.nlm.nih.gov/pubmed/10174663

7. Wetzel MS, Eisenberg DM, Kaptchuk TJ Courses involving complementary and alternative medicine at US medical schools. JAMA. 1998 Sep 2; 280(9):784-7. https://www.ncbi.nlm.nih.gov/pubmed/9729989

8. Virginia S Cowen1 and Vicki Cyr2.Complementary and alternative medicine in US medical schools. Published online 2015 Feb 12. doi: 10.2147/AMEP.S69761.PMCID: PMC4334197. . https://www.ncbi.nlm.nih.gov/pmc/articles/PMC4334197/

9. Kessler RC, Davis RB, Foster DF, Van Rompay MI, Walters EE, Wilkey SA, Kaptchuk TJ, Eisenberg DM Ann Intern Med. 2001 Aug 21; 135(4):262-8. Long-term trends in the use of complementary and alternative medical therapies in the United States. https://www.ncbi.nlm.nih.gov/pubmed/11511141

10. Fisher P, Ward A. Complementary medicine in Europe. BMJ. 1994 Jul 9; 309(6947):107-11. https://www.ncbi.nlm.nih.gov/pubmed/8038643

11. MacLennan AH, Wilson DH, Taylor AW. Prevalence and cost of alternative medicine in Australia. Lancet. 1996 Mar 2; 347(9001):569-73. https://www.ncbi.nlm.nih.gov/pubmed/8596318

12. London, UK: Mintel; 1997. Report on complementary medicines. https://www.emeraldinsight.com/doi/abs/10.1108/02634501011041462?mobileUi=0&journalCode=mip

13. Reverse Gut Diseases Naturally. http://michelle-honda-blog.renewyou.ca/crohns-colitis-book/

Chapter 10

1. Chandrasekhar K1, Kapoor J, Anishetty S. A prospective, randomized double-blind, placebo-controlled study of safety and efficacy of a high-concentration full-spectrum extract of ashwagandha root in reducing stress and anxiety in adults. Indian J Psychol Med. 2012 Jul;34(3):255-62. doi: 10.4103/0253-7176.106022. https://www.ncbi.nlm.nih.gov/pubmed/23439798

2. Cooley K1, Szczurko O, Perri D, Mills EJ, Bernhardt B, Zhou Q, Seely D.Naturopathic care for anxiety: a randomized controlled trial ISRCTN78958974. PLoS One. 2009 Aug 31;4(8):e6628. doi: 10.1371/journal.pone.0006628. https://www.ncbi.nlm.nih.gov/pubmed/19718255

3. Andrade C1, Aswath A, Chaturvedi SK, Srinivasa M, Raguram R. A double-blind, placebo-controlled evaluation of the anxiolytic efficacy of an ethanolic extract of withania somnifera.

    Indian J Psychiatry. 2000 Jul;42(3):295-301. https://www.ncbi.nlm.nih.gov/pubmed/21407960

4.   Candelario M1, Cuellar E1, Reyes-Ruiz JM2, Darabedian N3, Feimeng Z3, Miledi R2, Russo-Neustadt A1, Limon A4.Direct evidence for GABAergic activity of Withania somnifera on mammalian ionotropic GABAA and GABA receptors. J Ethnopharmacol. 2015 Aug 2;171:264-72. doi: 10.1016/j.jep.2015.05.058. Epub 2015 Jun 9. https://www.ncbi.nlm.nih.gov/pubmed/26068424

5.   Chandrasekhar K1, Kapoor J, Anishetty S. A prospective, randomized double-blind, placebo-controlled study of safety and efficacy of a high-concentration full-spectrum extract of ashwagandha root in reducing stress and anxiety in adults. https://www.ncbi.nlm.nih.gov/pubmed/23439798

6.   NUTRITION Evidence Based.Ashwagandha Dosage: How Much Should You Take per Day? https://www.healthline.com/nutrition/ashwagandha-dosage#stress-and-anxiety

7.   Holy Basil: Benefits for Your Brain and Your Body – Healthline. https://www.healthline.com/health/food-nutrition/basil-benefits

8.   Holy Basil: Uses, Side Effects, Interactions, Dosage, and Warning. https://www.webmd.com/vitamins/ai/ingredientmono-1101/holy-basil

9.   How the Placebo Effect Works in Psychology. Kendra Cherry. https://www.verywellmind.com/what-is-the-placebo-effect-2795466

10.   Rhodiola Rosea for Depression. https://www.medicalnewstoday.com/articles/319619.php

11.   The Calming Effects of Passionflower. https://www.healthline.com/health/anxiety/calming-effects-of-passionflower#calming

12.   Miyasaka LS, Atallah AN, Soares B. Passiflora for anxiety disorder. Cochrane Database of Systematic Reviews. 2007;(1):CD004518 [edited 2009]. http://www.thecochranelibrary.com

13.   How Is Passion Flower Used to Treat Anxiety? Verywell Mind. Mar 27, 2017. https://www.verywellmind.com/how-is-passion-flower-used-to-treat-anxiety-3024970

14.   Geller SE1, Studee L. Botanical and dietary supplements for mood and anxiety in menopausal women. 2007 May-Jun;14(3 Pt 1):541-9. https://www.ncbi.nlm.nih.gov/pubmed/17194961

15.   Skullcap - Wolfson, P. and D. L. Hoffmann. (2002).Alternative Therapies in Health and Medicine 9(2), 74-78) https://www.ncbi.nlm.nih.gov/pubmed/12652886

16.   Dr Stephen Gascoigne.Depression – gentle herbs that help. September, 2011. https://www.naturalhealthnews.uk/article/depression-%E2%80%93-herbal-remedies-that-help/

17. Seungyeop Lee and Dong-Kwon Rhee. Effects of ginseng on stress-related depression, anxiety, and the hypothalamic–pituitary–adrenal axis. Journal ListJ Ginseng Resv.41(4); 2017 OctPMC5628357.J Ginseng Res. 2017 Oct; 41(4): 589–594.Published online 2017 Jan 24. doi: 10.1016/j.jgr.2017.01.010. https://www.ncbi.nlm.nih.gov/pmc/articles/PMC5628357/

18. Le Fevre M., Matheny J., Kolt G.S. Eustress, distress, and interpretation in occupational stress. J Managerial Psychol. 2003;18:726–744. https://www.scirp.org/(S(351jmbntvnsjt1aadkposzje))/reference/ReferencesPapers.aspx?ReferenceID=1845215

19. Attele A.S., Wu J.A., Yuan C.S. Ginseng pharmacology: multiple constituents and multiple actions. Biochem Pharmacol. 1999;58:1685–1693. https://www.ncbi.nlm.nih.gov/pmc/articles/PMC2893180/

20. Kim D.H. Chemical diversity of Panax ginseng, Panax quinquifolium, and Panax notoginseng. J Ginseng Res. 2012;36:1–15. https://onlinelibrary.wiley.com/doi/full/10.1111/j.1527-3458.2007.00023.x

21. Liao B., Newmark H., Zhou R. Neuroprotective effects of ginseng total saponin and ginsenosides Rb1 and Rg1 on spinal cord neurons in vitro. Exp Neurol. 2002;173:224–234. https://www.ncbi.nlm.nih.gov/pmc/articles/PMC2808608/

22. Lee E., Kim S., Chung K.C., Choo M.K., Kim D.H., Nam G., Rhim H. 20(S)-Ginsenoside Rh2, a newly identified active ingredient of ginseng, inhibits NMDA receptors in cultured rat hippocampal neurons. Eur J Pharmacol. 2006;536:69–77. https://www.ncbi.nlm.nih.gov/pmc/articles/PMC3659517/

23. Thatte U., Bagadey S., Dahanukar S. Modulation of programmed cell death by medicinal plants. Cell Mol Biol. 2000;46:199–214. https://www.ncbi.nlm.nih.gov/pubmed/10726985

24. Ginseng. https://www.drugs.com/npp/ginseng.html

25. Mi Kyung Pyo,1,# Sun-Hye Choi,2,# Tae-Joon Shin,2,# Sung Hee Hwang. A Simple Method for the Preparation of Crude Gintonin from Ginseng Root, Stem, and Leaf. J Ginseng Res. 2011 Jun; 35(2): 209–218. https://www.ncbi.nlm.nih.gov/pmc/articles/PMC3659522/

26. Schisandra Berries – Great for Stress, Inflammation, Depression,Posted on June 21, 2017 by Dr. Paul Haider. https://paulhaider.wordpress.com/2017/06/21/schisandra-berries-great-for-stress-inflammation-depression/

27. Hattesohl M1, Feistel B, Sievers H, Lehnfeld R, Hegger M, Winterhoff H. Extracts of Valeriana officinalis L. s.l. show anxiolytic and antidepressant effects but neither sedative nor myorelaxant properties.

Phytomedicine. 2008 Jan;15(1-2):2-15. https://www.ncbi.nlm.nih.gov/pubmed/18160026

28.   Herbal Remedies for Depression and Anxiety - Mental Health Food. https://mentalhealthfood.net/13-herbs-for-treating-depression-and-anxiety/

29.   Natural Remedy for Anxiety and Depression Found in a Cup of Tea. UHN STAFF • NOV 14, 2015. https://universityhealthnews.com/daily/depression/natural-remedy-for-anxiety-found-in-a-cup-of-tea/

30.   Miyasaka LS, Atallah ÁN, Soares B. Valerian for anxiety disorders. Cochrane Database of Systematic Reviews. 2006;(4):CD004515 [edited 2009]. http://www.thecochranelibrary.com

31.   Kennedy DO, Scholey AB, Tildesley NT, Perry EK, Wesnes KA. Modulation of mood and cognitive performance following acute administration of Melissa officinalis (lemon balm). Pharmacol Biochem Behav. 2002 Jul;72(4):953-64. https://www.ncbi.nlm.nih.gov/pubmed/15378679

32.   How to Take Lemon Balm (Melissa officinalis). https://examine.com/supplements/melissa-officinalis/

33.   Anxiety: The Integrative Mental Health Solution, by James Lake MD. Oct 08, 2017. http://theintegrativementalhealthsolution.com/anxiety-the-integrative-mental-health-soution.html

34.   Can You Manage Bipolar Disorder Without Medication. https://www.healthyplace.com/.../can-you-manage-bipolar-disorder-without-medication

Chapter 11

1.   Phenylalanine. https://en.wikipedia.org/wiki/Phenylalanine

2.   Ji Hyun Ko1, Antonio P. Strafella. Dopaminergic Neurotransmission in the Human Brain: New Lessons from Perturbation and Imaging. Neuroscientist. 2012 Apr; 18(2): 149–168. https://www.ncbi.nlm.nih.gov/pmc/articles/PMC3479149/

3.   The FASEB Journal • http://www.tritolonen.fi/files/pdf/Patrick%20Ames%20part%202.pdf

4.   Vitamin D and the omega-3 fatty acids control serotonin synthesis and action. https://www.ncbi.nlm.nih.gov/pubmed/25713056

5.   Patrick, R. P., Ames, B. N. Vitamin D and the omega-3 fatty acids control serotonin synthesis and action, part 2: relevance for ADHD, bipolar, schizophrenia, and impulsive behavior. FASEB J. 29, 000–000 (2015). www.fasebj.org

6.	What is a normal estradiol level for a postmenopausal woman? https://www.breastcancer.org/tips/menopausal/types/determine-status

7.	Sharma, V., Khan, M., Corpse, C., and Sharma, P. (2008) Missed bipolarity and psychiatric comorbidity in women with postpartum depression. Bipolar Disord. 10, 742–747. https://www.ncbi.nlm.nih.gov/pmc/articles/PMC3961475/

8.	Sacher, J., Wilson, A. A., Houle, S., Rusjan, P., Hassan, S., Bloomfield, P. M., Stewart, D. E., and Meyer, J. H. (2010). Elevated brain monoamine oxidase A binding in the early postpartum period. Arch. Gen. Psychiatry 67, 468–474. https://www.ncbi.nlm.nih.gov/pmc/articles/PMC4443957/

9.	Dror, D. K., and Allen, L. H. (2010) Vitamin D inadequacy in pregnancy: biology, outcomes, and interventions. Nutr. Rev. 68,465–477. http://www.aipro.info/drive/File/Review_of_inadequency_of_vitamin_D_during_pregnancy_-_Aug_2010.pdf

10.	Maurizio Fava MD, David Mischoulon MD, PhD. Folate in Depression: Efficacy, Safety, Differences in Formulations and Clinical Issues. https://pdfs.semanticscholar.org/da67/41f63dbdcc1148f66afa69b-559c00dd49e75.pdf

11.	Papakostas GI, Shelton RC, Zajecka JM, Etemad B, Rickels K, & Clain A, et al. (2012). L-methylfolate as adjunctive therapy for SSRI-resistant major depression: results of two randomized, double-blind, parallel-sequential trials. American Journal of Psychiatry. 169(12), 1267-74. https://www.ncbi.nlm.nih.gov/pubmed/23212058

12.	Fluitt, N. (2012). L-Methylfolate: Another weapon against depression. Current Psychiatry, 11(1):72-72. https://www.mdedge.com/psychiatry/article/64587/depression/l-methylfolate-another-weapon-against-depression

13.	Johns Hopkins: Anemia of Folate Deficiency. http://www.hopkinsmedicine.org/healthlibrary/conditions/hematology_and_blood_disorders/anemia_of_folate_deficiency_85,P00089/

14.	Medical and Pharmacy Editor: John P. Cunha, DO, FACOEP. https://www.rxlist.com/consumer_lithium_eskalith_lithobid/drugs-condition.htm

15.	Dr. Richard A. Friedman. Professor of Psychiatry at Weill Cornell Medical College in Manhattan. September 25, 2012, on Page D6 of the New York edition with the headline: A Call for Caution on Antipsychotic Drugs. https://www.nytimes.com/2012/09/25/health/a-call-for-caution-in-the-use-of-antipsychotic-drugs.html

16.   Medscape. Lithium. https://reference.medscape.com/drug/eskalith-lithobid-lithium-342934

17.   Trace Mineral for Brain Health—Healing*Edge Sciences. www.healingedge.net/store/article_lithium_orotate.html

18.   Effects of lithium on cortical thickness and hippocampal subfield volumes in psychotic bipolar disorder C.I. Giakoumatos,a,b,1 P. Nanda,a,c,1 I.T. Mathew,a N. Tandon,a,d J. Shah,e,f J.R. Bishop,g B.A. Clementz,h,i G.D. Pearlson,j,k J.A. Sweeney,l C.A. Tamminga,l and M.S. Keshavana,m,* J Psychiatr Res. Author manuscript; available in PMC 2016 May 7. Published in final edited form as:J Psychiatr Res. 2015 Feb; 61: 180–187. Published online 2014 Dec 23. Doi: 10.1016/j.jpsychires.2014.12.008. https://www.ncbi.nlm.nih.gov/pmc/articles/PMC4859940/

19.   Fornai, F., et al., Autophagy and amyotrophic lateral sclerosis: The multiple roles of lithium. Autophagy, 2008. 4(4): p. 527-30. https://www.ncbi.nlm.nih.gov/pubmed/18367867

20.   Noble, W., et al., Inhibition of glycogen synthase kinase-3 by lithium correlates with reduced 6 tauopathy and degeneration in vivo. Proc Natl Acad Sci U S A, 2005. 102(19): p. 6990-5. https://www.ncbi.nlm.nih.gov/pubmed/15867159

21.   Can lithium or valproate untie tangles in Alzheimer's disease? Tariot PN, Aisen PS. J Clin Psychiatry. 2009 Jun; 70(6):919-21. https://www.ncbi.nlm.nih.gov/pubmed/19573485

22.   Review Lithium: potential therapeutics against acute brain injuries and chronic neurodegenerative diseases. Wada A, Yokoo H, Yanagita T, Kobayashi H. J Pharmacol Sci. 2005 Dec; 99(4):307-21. https://www.ncbi.nlm.nih.gov/pubmed/24398724

23.   A Lithium Orotate. Lithium (as Orotate) is a trace mineral that is Neuro-Protective and more. Healing Edge. www.healingedge.net/store/article_lithium_orotate.html

24.   Ann Jones: Lithium Aspartate Vs. Lithium Orotate: Aug 14, 2017. https://www.livestrong.com/article/519437-what-foods-contain-lithium/

25.   What Foods Contain Lithium? Andrea Cespedes. Updated: Oct 03, 2017 Livestrong.com. https://www.livestrong.com/article/519437-what-foods-contain-lithium/

26.   Balon, R., Possible dangers of a "nutritional supplement" lithium orotate. Ann Clin Psychiatry, 2013. 25(1): p. 71. https://www.alzdiscovery.org/cognitive-vitality/ratings/lithium-dietary

27.   By Maja Stanojevic, MD and Joe Cohen February 9, 2014.Top 23 Lithium Orotate Benefits + Side Effects & Toxicity. Reviewed by Jonathan

Ritter, PharmD, PhD (Pharmacology) https://selfhacked.com/blog/the-benefits-of-lithium/

28. S-Adenosylmethionine (SAMe) for Neuropsychiatric Disorders: A Clinician-Oriented Review of Research.Anup Sharma, MD, PhD,1 Patricia Gerbarg, MD,2 Teodoro Bottiglieri, PhD,3 Lila Massoumi, MD,4 Linda L. Carpenter, MD,5 Helen Lavretsky, MD,6 Philip R. Muskin, MD,7 Richard P. Brown, MD,7 and David Mischoulon, MD, PhD8. J Clin Psychiatry. 2017 Jun; 78(6): e656–e667. https://www.ncbi.nlm.nih.gov/pmc/articles/PMC5501081/

29. A Teodoro Bottiglieri at Baylor Scott & White Health. Biochemical Study of Depressed Patients Receiving S-Adenosyl-L-Methionine (SAM). Chapter from book Biological Methylation and Drug Design: Experimental and Clinical Role of S-Adenosylmethionine (pp.327-338). https://www.researchgate.net/publication/279405916_A_Biochemical_Study_of_Depressed_Patients_Receiving_S-Adenosyl-L-Methionine_SAM

30. 33. Richard P. Brown, M.D. Investigating SAM-e for Depression. http://arthusbio.com/wp-content/uploads/2018/10/20.pdf

31. M.De Vanna1R.Rigamonti2. Oral S-adenosyl-L-methionine in depression. Current Therapeutic Research. Volume 52, Issue 3, September 1992, Pages 478-485. https://www.sciencedirect.com/science/article/pii/S0011393X05804242

32. Magnesium Might Boost Mood | Psychology Today. Sep 26, 2017. https://www.psychologytoday.com/us/blog/open-gently/.../magnesium-might-boost-mood

33. Association between magnesium intake and depression and anxiety in community-dwelling adults: the Hordaland Health Study Felice N. Jacka, Simon Overland, Robert Stewart, Grethe S. Tell, Ingvar Bjelland & Arnstein Mykletun Pages 45-52 | Received 17 Sep 2008, Published online: 06 Jul 2009. https://www.tandfonline.com/doi/abs/10.1080/00048670802534408

34. ACTH Hormone Test: Purpose, Procedure, and Results – Healthline. Sep 22, 2017. https://www.healthline.com/health/acth

35. Szewczyk B1, Kubera M, Nowak G. The role of zinc in neurodegenerative inflammatory pathways in depression. Prog Neuropsychopharmacol Biol Psychiatry. 2011 Apr 29;35(3):693-701. doi: 10.1016/j.pnpbp.2010.02.010. Epub 2010 Feb 13. https://www.ncbi.nlm.nih.gov/pubmed/20156515 .

36. Emily Deans, M.D. Zinc: an Antidepressant. Evolutionary Psychiatry. Sep 15, 2013. https://www.psychologytoday.com/ca/blog/evolutionary-psychiatry/201309/zinc-antidepressant

37.   Stunning Benefits of MCT Oil. Joan Clark. https://www.tipsbulletin.com/mct-oil-benefits/

38.   Courchesne-Loyer A., Fortier M., Tremblay-Mercier J., Chouinard-Watkins R., Roy M., Nugent S., et al. (2013). Stimulation of mild, sustained ketonemia by medium-chain triacylglycerols in healthy humans: estimated potential contribution to brain energy metabolism. Nutrition 29 635–640. 10.1016/j.nut.2012.09.009. https://www.ncbi.nlm.nih.gov/pubmed/23274095

39.   Phosphatidylserine: Uses and Risks - WebMD. https://www.webmd.com/vitamins-and-supplements/phosphatidylserine-uses-and-risks

40.   Why Phosphatidylserine May Be The Answer to Stress, ADHD, Depression, Anxiety & Insomnia. https://perfectketo.com/phosphatidylserine/

41.   Phosphatidylserine: Why You Should Include it in Your Diet. https://neurohacker.com/phosphatidylserine-why-you-should-include-it-in-your-diet

42.   Shrinivas K. Kulkarni, Mohit Kumar, Bhutani Mahendra Bishnoi. Antidepressant activity of curcumin: involvement of serotonin and dopamine system. December 2008, 201:435. https://link.springer.com/article/10.1007/s00213-008-1300-y

43.   Akazawa N1, Choi Y, Miyaki A, Tanabe Y, Sugawara J, Ajisaka R, Maeda S. Curcumin ingestion and exercise training improve vascular endothelial function in postmenopausal women. Nutr Res. 2012 Oct;32(10):795-9. https://www.ncbi.nlm.nih.gov/pubmed/23146777

44.   Study Shows Turmeric Can Reduce Symptoms of Depression, Anxiety. Journal of Affective Disorders 167(2014)368-375. https://www.prnewswire.com/news-releases/study-shows-turmeric-can-reduce-symptoms-of-depression-anxiety-546535422.html

45.   On the Neuroprotective Role of Astaxanthin: New Perspectives? Christian Galasso,1 Ida Orefice,1 Paola Pellone,1 Paola Cirino,2 Roberta Miele,1 Adrianna Ianora,1 Christophe Brunet,1,* and Clementina Sansone1, Mar Drugs. 2018 Aug; 16(8): 247. https://www.ncbi.nlm.nih.gov/pmc/articles/PMC6117702/

Chapter 12

1.   Environ Health Perspect. 2002 Jun. 110 Suppl 3:349-53.Goitrogenic and estrogenic activity of soy isoflavones. Doerge DR1, Sheehan DM. https://www.ncbi.nlm.nih.gov/pubmed/12060828

2.   Biochem Pharmacol. 1997 Nov 15;54(10):1087-96. Anti-thyroid isoflavones from soybean: isolation, characterization, and mechanisms of

action. Divi RL1, Chang HC, Doerge DR. https://www.ncbi.nlm.nih.gov/pubmed/9464451

3. The Antidepressant Effect of L-Tyrosine-Loaded Nanoparticles: Behavioral Aspects. Alabsi A1, Khoudary AC1, Abdelwahed W2. https://www.ncbi.nlm.nih.gov/pubmed/27647959

4. Meyers S. Use of neurotransmitter precursors for treatment of depression. Altern Med Rev. 2000;5(1):64-71 https://www.ncbi.nlm.nih.gov/pubmed/10696120

5. Abdelrahman Alabsi, Adel Charbel Khoudary, Wassim Abdelwahed, The Antidepressant Effect of L-Tyrosine-Loaded Nanoparticles: Behavioral Aspects. Ann Neurosci 2016 Jul 7;23(2):89-99.Epub 2016 Jul 7. https://www.ncbi.nlm.nih.gov/pmc/articles/PMC5020390/

6. The Path to Phenomenal Health Sam Graci 2005; 119. Retrieved Nov. 2016. http://www.vitasource365.com/the-path-to-phenomenal-health-by-sam-graci.html

7. American Thyroid Association, Iodine Deficiency. http://www.thyroid.org/iodine-deficiency/

8. International Council for the Control of Iodine Deficiency Disorders. http://www.iccidd.org

9. Iodine Status Worldwide, WHO Global Database on Iodine Deficiency, Geneva 2004. http://apps.who.int/iris/bitstream/10665/43010/1/9241592001.pdf

10. Bernecker C. Acta Allergol. 1969 Sep;24(3):216-25. Intermittent therapy with potassium iodide in chronic obstructive disease of the airways. A review of 10 years' experience. http://www.ncbi.nlm.nih.gov/pubmed/5395878

11. Kent Hoftorf M.D., Thyroid Blood Tests Don't Always Tell the Whole Story. April 6, 2012 https://www.holtorfmed.com/ and https://www.nahypothyroidism.org/thyroid-blood-tests-dont-always-tell-the-whole-story/

12. "How Accurate is TSH Testing?" NAHypothyroidism.org. Retrieved 2019-2-26. https://www.nahypothyroidism.org/how-accurate-is-tsh-testing/

13. A fact sheet on Adrenal Insufficiency can be found online at: www.hormone.org/Resources/upload/adrenal-insufficiency-bilingual-081810.pdf

14. Mousumi Bose, Blanca Oliván, and Blandine Laferrère. Curr Opin Endocrinol Diabetes Obes. 2009 Oct; 16(5): 340–346.doi: 10.1097/MED.0b013e32832fa137. (weight gain) https://www.ncbi.nlm.nih.gov/pmc/articles/PMC2858344/

15. Betterle C, Morlin L. Autoimmune Addison's disease. In: Ghizzoni L, Cappa M, Chrousos G, Loche S, Maghnie M, eds. Pediatric Adrenal Diseases. Endocrine Development. Vol. 20. Padova, Italy: Karger Publishers; 2011: 161–172. Adrenal Insufficiency & Addison's Disease, What is adrenal insufficiency? https://www.niddk.nih.gov/health-information/endocrine-diseases/adrenal-insufficiency-addisons-disease

16. Dr. Nikolas Hedberg, Supplements that Help Correct Adrenal Dysfunction-Thyroid Adrenal Pancreas Axis' Sep 18, 2016. http://drhedberg.com/herbal-medicines-for-thyroid-disorders/